Acclaim

"An intimate reflection on one wise woman's medical journey from symptom to recovery. This book relates how Marilyn Hagar turned to her trusted inner guides, her dreams and her art, to support her when her life was radically disrupted with an illness. She inspires us to access our inner healer when faced with challenges, and reminds us that when dealing with chaotic times, we can't hold on to a frozen notion of who we think we are or how we think things should be. In her words, 'Better to open to the creative power deep inside and listen to our instincts and intuitions about what is trying to emerge.'"
    —Joan Stanford, poet, art therapist, and author of *The Art of Play: Ignite Your Imagination to Unlock Insight, Healing, and Joy*

"I was deeply moved by *The Scalpel, the Paintbrush, and the Pen*, a story of healing that is full of wisdom, courage, and heart. Marilyn's truth-telling and self-reflection on her experiences illustrate that our individual paths through illness and treatment are mythic healing journeys on which we can discover resources deep within ourselves as we partner with the helpers we encounter along the way."
    —Mary Cavagnaro, poet, psychotherapist

The Scalpel, the Paintbrush, and the Pen

Healing as a Creative Art

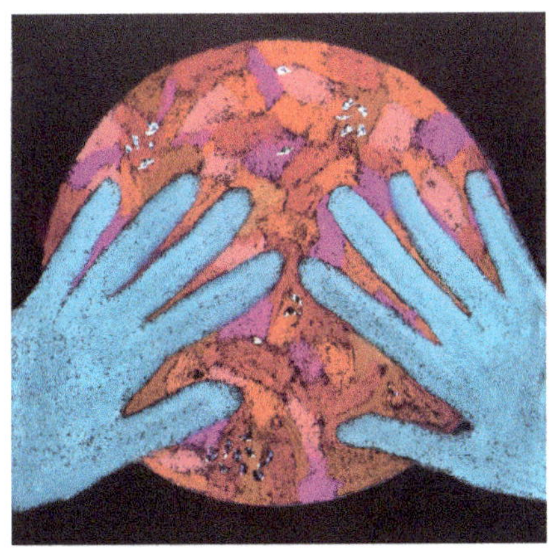

By

Marilyn Kay Hagar

Wild Inside Books
Mendocino

Wild Inside Books
42341 Little Lake Road
Mendocino, CA 95460
marilynhagar.com

Cover design: Allegra Pescatore
Book Production: Cypress House

"The Old Woman of the World" from *Why the World Doesn't End: Tales of Renewal in Times of Loss* used by permission of Michael J. Meade (copyright © 2012, GreenFire Press).

"The Breeze at Dawn" from *The Essential Rumi,* copyright ©1995, used by permission of Coleman Barks.

Print ISBN: 979-8-9882538-0-8
Ebook ISBN: 979-8-9882538-1-5

Publisher's Cataloging-in-Publication Data
Names: Hagar, Marilyn Kay, author.
Title: The scalpel, the paintbrush, and the pen : healing as a creative art / by
    Marilyn Kay Hagar.
Description: First edition. | Mendocino, [California] : Wild Inside Books,
    [2023]
Identifiers: ISBN: 979-8-9882538-0-8 (print) | 979-8-9882538-1-5 (ePub) |
    LCCN: 2023916164
Subjects: LCSH: Hagar, Marilyn Kay--Health. | Healing--Psychological
    aspects. | Self-consciousness (Awareness) | Mind and body. | Art therapy.
    | Dreams. | Intuition. | BISAC: HEALTH & FITNESS / Diseases & Condi-
    tions / Cancer.
Classification: LCC: R726.5 .H34 2023 | DDC: 615.5--dc23

Printed in the United States of America
2 4 6 8 9 7 5 3 1
First edition

*To Dr. Mohamed Abdelgidir Adam,
and to all of my family and all of my friends.
With deepest gratitude for your kind hearts and all of your help.
I wouldn't have made it through without you.*

Table of Contents

*The intuitive mind is a sacred gift and
the rational mind is a faithful servant.*
*We have created a society that honors the
servant and has forgotten the gift.*

—Albert Einstein

Before You Read My Story

Sometimes the most ordinary moments stay with us for a lifetime. They stay because they've reached down inside us and grabbed onto something essential. When we take note, these memories can shine a light into our future, helping us manifest our highest hopes and our biggest dreams.

I experienced one of those moments many years ago, and it touches my heart to this day. I was sitting on a beach in Maui with my young family. I watched as an elderly couple nearby struggled to their feet. Once upright, the two held hands and wobbled their way towards the water. I was self-conscious in my bathing suit, my stomach still protruding just six weeks after giving birth to my third son, but these old ones didn't seem to be a bit embarrassed about their wrinkled, out of shape bodies. Clad in old fashioned bathing suits, they laughed their way down to the surf. When the water puddled around their feet, they got down on their hands and knees and crawled out into the ocean. They were in hysterics each time a big wave rolled them back to the shore. Then they got back up on their hands and knees and challenged the ocean once again. I had never witnessed such a surrender to pure play in folks their age. I sat there nursing my infant son and vowed that when I got old, I wanted to be just like them.

Fast forward through many years, and I found myself in mid-life, divorced, children grown, living alone in my forest home where I had raised my family. This was not at all the life I had envisioned when I sat on the beach all those years ago. I had pledged to remain in my marriage "until death do us part," but just as our sons were in the process of leaving home, my husband left home as well. Life sent us down separate roads after twenty-five years of marriage.

I recreated myself at that time, envisioning a new dream for my life, one centered around my work as an expressive arts therapist. Rather than embarking on a career, I had found my calling. My work was intimately tied to my own search for meaning and purpose. I wanted to explore the depths of who we are as human beings and help myself and others discover the unique gifts we each have to offer to our world.

Our youthful hopes and dreams head us in a direction, but they often manifest in ways that are quite different from what we expected. Here I am now in old age. I am not part of an old couple, reflecting over all we have created in our years together, but I have found a life of meaning and purpose. Fulfilling that vow made on the beach in Maui long ago, I have indeed come to old age with an alive and playful spirit.

The ability to play as an adult is an important part of the story I will tell here. The twist that makes me different from those old ones I've so remembered is that I am diving deep into the waters of the unconscious mind, playing there in a multiplicity of ways and finding treasure in the depths of the human imagination.

Playing in the Imagination

In my first book, *Finding the Wild Inside, Exploring Our Inner Landscape Through the Arts, Dreams, and Intuition*, I told the story of how, with an awakened imagination, I learned to communicate with my inner world. I did this by playing in the arts and using them for self-reflection, exploring the symbolic language of my nightly dreams, and greeting synchronicities with awe and wonder. All of this broadened my access to my intuition. None of it would have happened had I not learned this important lesson: Playing in the realm of my imagination is as vital to my life now as it was when

I was a child. When I tell you my story, you will see how important that lesson became when my good health was suddenly challenged.

When I was young, my best friend Judy and I lived and breathed in a world of, "Let's pretend." We turned the swings in the schoolyard into rocket ships and imagined wild adventures in outer space. On other days we rode imaginary horses, rescued those in need, and made all the bad guys pay. The difference between that kind of child's play and the imaginative play I experience as an adult is that now I seek the meaning of what my imagination brings to the fore. Truly, our ability to imagine is one of the greatest gifts of being human. It is important that we nurture that part of ourselves. That, more than anything else, has helped to keep the magical child who believes anything is possible alive and well inside of me. I hold her in my heart. She is important to my story because being open to all possibilities goes hand in hand with being open to healing.

As you will learn in this book, a year after my first book came out, I was diagnosed with a life-threatening illness. It wasn't something that was going to kill me immediately but very troubling, none the less. This writing is about how I found and stayed in close communication with my own inner healer as I entered the medical world and made my way, step by step, on my healing journey. I was so grateful to have that magical child inside leading the way. While I was moving through what I called a healing crisis, she was on an adventure, playing, asking questions, exploring, making art, dreaming, and talking to foxes. All of this helped the adult me make meaning from all that I was experiencing, and that helped both of us make it through.

When Things Fall Apart

Life is not always expanding, it also contracts. Not one of us escapes moments when it feels like life as we know it has come to an end. That was certainly true for me when I received my medical diagnosis. When life turns us upside down like that, looking inside for our own deepest wisdom gives us ground to walk on. If you are facing disruption, I hope this book will be an inspiration. I guarantee that you, like all of us, have a wise one inside just waiting for you to begin a conversation. That conversation can lead to a deep relationship with part of you that you may have only glimpsed before. When I looked inside in this way, I met a part of myself that I didn't even know existed. Now, she guides my life.

As I tell my story in this book, I have included the artwork I did throughout my healing journey. I also share some important dreams. I talk about what both my drawings and my dreams mean to me, how they speak to me, and how that helped me along my way. It might surprise you to know that no talent or skill is necessary to learn from the inner practices that are part of my story. They are available to all of us simply because we are human. I hope as you see how I used these gifts to help me through my healing journey, you might be inspired to open to them as well. If you are already using them, I urge you to continue. There is no end to exploration in these realms. The Now It's Your Turn section at the end of my book will direct you to my website where I offer experiences based on major themes in each chapter of this book. You might want to look there as you read along.

What I desperately needed when life fell apart was some ease with the falling apart itself. As a member of a culture that worships youth and likes to believe in the possibility of unbounded growth and expansion, I had to learn through confrontation with dissolution that sometimes things fall away. My divorce was my first big lesson in the death of something I had put my whole heart into. When illness came into my life, I had to find a whole new tolerance for life's unravelling.

I feel lucky that in the years before my diagnosis I had been caring for my elderly parents. Those years of caregiving allowed me a peek into the dissolution awaiting us at the far end of life. My father died in his sleep at 94, as did my mother at almost 102. No matter how dedicated we have been to caring for ourselves, in the end, life has a way of winding us down. In those last years with my parents, I learned oodles about life letting go of itself and the beauty of embracing this final phase of our existence.

As I entered old age myself, I began focusing my work on issues of aging, leading groups and workshops on that theme. My friend and colleague Joan Stanford, author of *The Art of Play, Ignite Your Imagination to Unlock Insight, Healing and Joy,* and I were embracing the archetype of the Crone, the third phase of the Triple Goddess, in our teachings.

We discovered an old folk myth that Michael Meade recounts in his book, *Why the World Doesn't End.* The old story touches on the theme of life unravelling and is a deep teaching about how to proceed when that happens. Before I introduce you further to this book and my story, I want to invite you to use your imagination and come with me to pay a visit to the Old Woman of the World.

The Old Woman of the World

If you are willing, pause for a moment and take some deep breaths. If it feels right, imagine your younger self snuggled up beside you, ready to listen to this ancient tale. When you feel ready, step with me into her cave. You will see her there, sitting in her chair doing her important work. She is weaving, and she wants to make the most beautiful garment in the whole wide world. Weaving has been absorbing her energy for a very long time, and what she is creating is nearing completion.

As we watch, she is working on the fringed edge of her garment. She wants to weave it with porcupine quills because she knows that the things that poke us in life are also things of beauty. She wants to weave that important message into this beautiful garment.

Aside from weaving, the old woman has another job that occupies her time. In the very back of the cave a soup is bubbling in a cauldron. The cauldron sits over a flame that is so old no one can recall its beginning. The soup contains all the things that grow on the earth, and it must be stirred occasionally, so those precious things don't become scorched or burned. The Old Woman of the World understands the necessity of each of her jobs. She is in sync with the big energies in the world and knows when she needs to weave things together and when she needs to stir things up.

In your mind's eye, watch now as she lays her beautiful weaving on the floor and makes her way to the back of the cave where the cauldron bubbles, waiting to be tended. We aren't the only ones watching. A black dog lives in that cave with the old woman. While he may have been sleeping, his head pops up now, as he sees the old woman walking away. When she is fully occupied stirring that pot at the back of the cave, he gets up, walks over, and begins to play with the that beautiful garment. See now how he finds a loose thread and pulls on it with his sharp teeth. As the black dog pulls, the garment begins to unravel, and by the time the old woman returns, she finds her weaving destroyed, now a chaotic mess of loose threads and porcupine quills strewn across the floor of the cave.

The Old Woman stands quietly for some time, beholding this mess. Then watch as she bends down and picks up one single thread. With that thread, she begins her weaving all over again. As she weaves, the threads begin to reveal new images, and soon she is expanding on the patterns of the old weaving. New visions guide her now as she loses herself in creating this garment, excited once again to be creating the most beautiful garment in the whole wide world.

Take a moment now and reflect on your experience there in the cave watching the Old Woman. Is there a part of the story that stands out to you? Why do you think that is so? I wish for you that the next time the black dog visits your life, you can stand in the mess he makes and when you are ready, look for the thread that is yours to find. See where that thread wants to take you.

Finding Beauty in the Poke

Receiving my medical diagnosis was like a poke from one of the Old Woman's porcupine quills. It completely unraveled life as I knew it. The story I want to tell you in this book is about how I found the beauty in the poke, a beauty untouched by the daunting events of my healing journey or its outcome, a beauty that rests at the center of everything. That said, believe me there were plenty of days when I felt just like that Old Woman standing there surveying the mess. Now that I've found my way to recovery, writing this book is the thread I'm picking up as I begin reweaving myself back into the web that is life.

I call the time before my diagnosis "the before time." Back then, using the story of the Old Woman in the Cave in our work together, Joan and I had designed a group ritual and art process to honor moments of dissolution in our lives. We had airline tickets in hand and were ready to set off to present our workshop at the International Expressive Arts Therapy Conference when the Covid pandemic hit and brought our plans to a screeching halt. From one day to the next, we were all informed that life as we had known it was over. We were told to shelter in our homes, only going out for necessities. At first it seemed unreal. How could this be? Everything had stopped, everything! In the beginning I remember thinking that this was a temporary situation, but of course, it was not. The Old Woman was stirring the pot and the black dog was unraveling the weaving that was our lives.

When Joan and I next met, outdoors and socially distanced, we couldn't help but laugh. We felt like we had been students of unravelling, but even in our wildest imaginations, we wouldn't have predicted the extent of the dissolution we were living through, and it was worldwide!

History will have much to say about this time in our lives, but it seems important to mention it here because one year into the pandemic, before the vaccine became available, my medical problem revealed itself, ushering in a time of further unravelling, now on a deeply personal level. My outer life was already so altered that I didn't think that further dissolution was possible, but it certainly was. The world was in chaos, and so was I.

I expressed the chaos I was feeling in those times in this drawing which I titled, *The Unravelling.*

Receiving a scary medical diagnosis or living through a life-altering crisis of some other nature, sends us tumbling, like a baby bird, out of the nest where we felt safe and warm. Suddenly the world is cold and very big. We need new skills, as seemingly impossible as learning how to fly, to navigate to safety.

This book chronicles my journey in that new world where I found myself floundering in the shadow of the physicality of my disease. It wasn't long before I found sparks of light in that darkness. Those sparks lit my way and let me know that I was being held by an energy larger than my little ego self. I grew wings and I learned to fly. Each time I thought I might fall from the sky, I felt a strong current of air uplifting me. Though invisible, I came to trust that current.

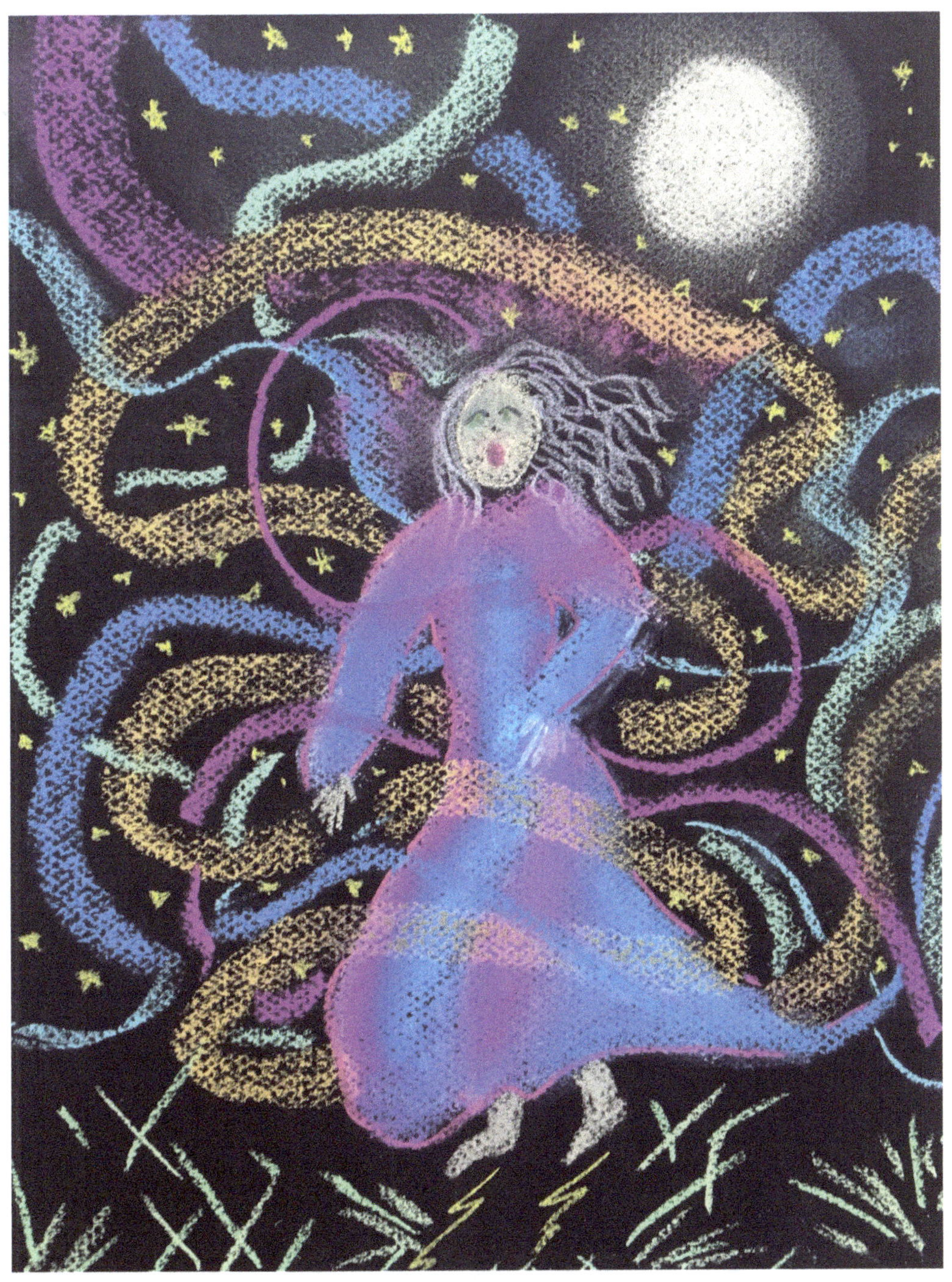

The Unravelling

We humans don't go on a journey like this without it changing us. Here I am, touching ground and wondering who I have become now. It's my hope that my journey will shed the light you need on yours. Whether like me, you are facing a life-threatening illness or whether you are experiencing some other kind of disruption, may you, too, grow wings and fly, coming through it all to touch the ground in a life filled with many new possibilities.

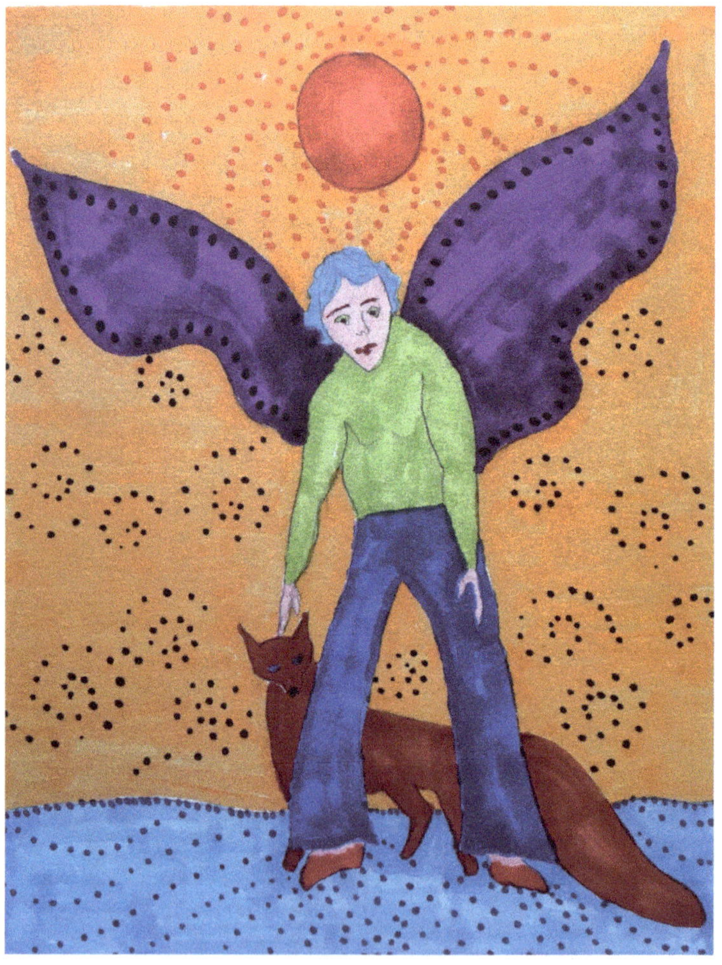

Touching Ground

Chapter 1

The Unravelling

It all started with a bloody tampon. Not mine, not even a real one, but a dream image shared by a young woman in a group I attend where we share our nightly dreams with one another and explore their possible meanings. When she spoke of the bloody tampon lying on the floor in her dream, my mind wandered. *Wow, women are still menstruating—that is all still going on,* I thought to myself. For me as an older woman, it seemed like eons since that was a regular part of my life.

Seeing the bloody tampon in my own imagination instantly brought back visceral memories of a younger time: that wet feeling between my legs, the deep red clots in the toilet, the metallic odor. Back then, my life cycled through time, my body tying me to the fecundity of wild nature. I don't think I honored that properly at the time, but looking back I missed living my life inside of those circles. Time in my later years feels more linear, less informed by natural cycles, especially as we reach old age. From that perspective, there is nowhere to go but the end of the line, and none of us like to think about that.

Our evening of dream sharing soon came to a close. We bid one another goodnight. I clicked off my computer as we had been meeting on Zoom. It was late and I was tired. I turned out the lights and went upstairs to ready myself for bed. Sitting on the toilet to pee one last time before I climbed into bed, I wiped myself, and there it was, blood on the toilet tissue.

"What? This can't be! I looked again in disbelief, but there it was—blood.

Sleep didn't come easy that night. A river of thoughts cascaded through my mind. As an expressive arts therapist, I had led a cancer support group in my town for a couple of years. I thought of those brave folks I'd met back then. Is this how it was for them at the beginning of it all? From one moment to the next, the boogeyman of ill health jumps out of nowhere and says *Boo!* In that single moment, you realize that something is profoundly wrong with you, and you witness your remarkably good health slip away before your very eyes.

I was afraid I was heading down that dark road, a road I'd never been down before. Pulling myself back to the present moment, I told myself I would call my doctor in the morning and hoped there was some easy explanation for the blood. As I drifted off to sleep, I thought about the woman's dream of a bloody tampon and my trip down memory lane that the image had evoked. Could the dream have triggered such a physical response in my body? I was certain that was not possible, but I wondered at the synchronicity of the shared dream and my own bloody event—was it portending something?

It was the darkest time of the year, just days before Christmas. Amazingly, I was able to get an appointment with Carla, a certified nurse midwife and family nurse practitioner who handles women's care at the clinic where I received my medical care. I had known Carla for years as our kids had gone to school together, but this was the first time I had gone to her as a patient. I felt I was in good hands.

My appointment was on the Winter Solstice. It was 2020, and the Covid pandemic was raging, though we were just on the cusp of being able to be vaccinated. I'd been isolated at home for months, only going out every couple of weeks for necessities. I was afraid of being exposed to the virus as I entered the medical clinic, but I put on my mask and hoped for the best. In the beginning, I was optimistic that all would turn out okay, as it always had. Carla didn't seem terribly alarmed about my situation. She didn't find anything ominous in my physical examination, but she wanted me to have an ultrasound of my pelvis to look into it further. That day, all the testing and the nerve-wracking waiting for results began.

I had the ultrasound procedure and was waiting patiently to hear what the results might tell us. Eli, the youngest of my three sons, and his wife Amy had arrived to celebrate Christmas with me a couple of days early at my home in Mendocino, California. They had driven the three hours down from Eureka in northern California where they lived. We visited outside on the deck, so as not to expose one another to the virus. That afternoon I received a phone call from Carla telling me that the ultrasound showed a pelvic mass. I felt a numbness fall over me. When I hung up the phone, I sat for a moment trying to let this information find some kind of comfortable place in me before I rejoined my company. Not able to do that, I walked back out on the deck as if through a dense fog and told Eli and Amy what I had just learned.

It was lovely to be with family as my health news darkened. We barbequed our dinner outside in the middle of winter, laughing at our boldness, and climbed into down sleeping bags when it got too cold to visit comfortably. I felt as if I were living in two realities, one full of the warmth and comfort of family, and the other cold and gray, a big dark cloud looming over me.

I was afraid that impending storm was going to shatter life as I knew it; it could even end it.

Carla ordered blood tests and a CT scan for further diagnosis. It was Christmas Eve morning when they took my blood and sent it off for analysis. I knew the blood tests were cancer markers used to diagnose ovarian cancer. That was scary, but I was still optimistic, thinking that the mass could be benign. I was so used to my body working as it was meant to, I had trouble absorbing the fact that something might be seriously wrong. After all, there was only that one sighting of blood. I'd had no further symptoms.

When my family left later that day, I found myself sinking more deeply into my fear about what was happening to me. I calmed myself with my rational mind, telling myself I would just have to go step by step through this until things were clearer. But that night when I went to bed, my body began to tremble, literally to shake uncontrollably with fear. I felt like a small child cowering in the face of a force more powerful than anything I had encountered before. As my body was letting me know just how frightened I really was, the denial about my situation began to fade, and the fog that had descended around me begin to clear. I realized I could recognize my fear and still move forward. *Isn't that the definition of courage?* I asked myself.

An Unexpected Gift

It was stormy when I woke up on Christmas morning. Despite the weather, I was determined to go for my dawn walk on the headlands that surround my town. I bundled myself up in my rain gear and set out. It was blustery, with winds whipping about so powerfully that I had to watch my balance as I walked along the cliffs overlooking the ocean. Dark clouds tumbled in the sky overhead, and before long I was walking in pouring rain.

There was no one else on the headlands that morning, but there was nowhere else I would rather be. The storm mirrored my inner reality. It was as if I were in sync with the world. The words of that old song, "When you walk through a storm, hold your head up high and don't be afraid of the dark," began singing inside my mind. I was energized by this storm, proud of myself for being out there despite it all. I could have stayed in bed that cold morning, but this walk was giving me a surprise Christmas gift, one I didn't know I was asking for.

The ravens were effortlessly floating on the air currents, the ocean was roaring, the waves were crashing onto the rocks below. In an ecstatic moment, I felt the energy of wild nature supporting me in every possible way. It was as if Mother Nature were holding me in her hand. Tears came when I heard a voice from deep inside: *Marilyn, this is all going to be okay. Whatever happens, you will be able to deal with it.* In that moment, every part of me realized it was true. Even if this turned out to be a worst-case scenario and these events were the harbinger of my death, I would be able to deal with it. I was overwhelmed with gratitude for everything that had happened to me in my life, for everything and everyone who had helped me come to this precious realization. My tears that morning were not coming from a place of struggle but rather from a place of grace. This was the first of many moments to come when I found myself filled with deep peace in the midst of my stormy medical situation.

Because of the holiday, it was a long wait for the blood test results to come back. When they did, they fell out of normal range—not terribly, but not right. Carla told me that her patients with ovarian cancer had numbers much higher than mine, but still mine were not normal and we needed to look further. We'd see what the CT scan showed. There was still a question as to what all of this meant, but as each test came back with concerning results, my confidence that it was not a serious matter dwindled rapidly.

I had the CT scan just before the New Year's holiday, so there was another extra-long wait for the results. Each day felt like an eternity. Five days into the new year, Carla finally called with news. She told me there were areas on my ovaries that showed a bunch of tiny little circles on the scan. Those little circles were cysts. I was diagnosed with *adnexal cysts,* the medical terminology for fluid-filled cysts in the area of the pelvis around the uterus. She told me they could be benign, but the threat of ovarian cancer still loomed. She referred me to a gynecologist for further advice and follow up.

The earliest appointment with the gynecologist was a few weeks away, so there was more waiting in store for me. But before that meeting could take place, I received another call from Carla telling me that after looking at my scan, the gynecologist thought I would be better served at one of the larger medical centers in the Bay Area. That is how I found my way to the University of California San Francisco Medical Center at Mission Bay.

Surgery and A New Diagnosis

January had turned into February when I finally met with Dr. Chen, a surgeon at UCSF Medical Center's gynecologic oncology surgery department. She told me I was a good candidate for the surgery I would need to have, and that it could be done laparoscopically. This was good news because it meant that the surgery could be done making only a few half-inch incisions and so be easier to recover from than if done by one large incision. The plan was to do a partial hysterectomy, removing my affected ovaries. During the surgery, they would send tissue samples to the lab, and if there was any malignancy, I might have to have a complete hysterectomy.

My surgery was scheduled for February 18th. I celebrated receiving my first Covid vaccine shot before my surgery. It made me feel a little more comfortable about being in the hospital and going out into the world.

Eli drove down from Eureka, picked me up, and drove me to San Francisco, an additional 3-hour drive south. In control of his own work schedule as a consulting aquatic ecologist, Eli was able to take time away from his job. His wife Amy fully supported my son coming to help me, telling me she was glad he could be of support. It is what she would want to do for her own parents if either of them was ever in my situation. Still, I felt that his coming to help disrupted their lives and was in that sense, a sacrifice for both of them.

We stayed in a motel in Marin County the night before the surgery, which meant more exposure to Covid. Having had only one Covid shot, I was worried for myself, but I was more worried for Eli who at 43 hadn't yet qualified for the vaccine. Such times we were living in! At that time, we still thought Covid was possibly spread on surfaces (turns out it is but very minimally; it spreads more dominantly through respiratory droplets). Motels were turning themselves inside out to prove it would be safe to stay, advertising windows that could be opened and assuring that all surfaces would be carefully disinfected.

That next morning, we drove across the Golden Gate Bridge as the sun rose, and under that pink sky, Eli dropped me off at the hospital door. Due to the pandemic, no one but the patient was allowed to enter.

My surgery was supposed to be two hours long. It was possible that I would go home that same day, but when I came off the anesthesia, it was night. I was drugged and confused. As I floated in and out of sleep, a nurse told me that I would be spending the night. I told her that I was worried about my son.

"How old is your son?" the nurse asked me.

"Forty-three," I responded. She laughed, as did someone else who was in the room. They were probably thinking, *My God, do mothers never stop worrying about their children?* I drifted back into the dark cloud of anesthesia before I could explain my concern. *Where was he? Did he find a motel in the San Francisco area or go back to Marin? Was he safe? Had anyone told him what was happening to me?*

I was too out of it to remember my cell phone was right across the room in a bag with my belongings, and I could have called him myself. It was hard to be in the hospital without a loved one there to help me orient. Aside from what Eli knew, it remains unclear to me if I learned that night what had actually happened in the surgery.

As it turned out, I had to have a full hysterectomy. The tissue examined during surgery was not malignant, but there was another problem, one that originated in my appendix, not my ovaries. I was diagnosed with a condition called *low grade appendiceal mucinous neoplasms*, referred to as LAMN for short. A *mucinous neoplasm* is an abnormal and excessive growth of tissue that is filled with fluid, or *mucin.* Thus, all those tiny circles on my CT scan.

In my case, the neoplasms had begun growing inside my appendix. Without any noticeable symptoms, my appendix had opened, and the mucin escaped, seeding the growth of neoplasms in my abdominal cavity. My appendix had sealed itself back up, but now the neoplasms had spread and were flourishing on my ovaries. They were visible there, but the problem could be spreading microscopically, so even with a complete hysterectomy and the removal of my appendix, the neoplasms were now at home in my abdomen where they would continue to multiply.

LAMN is a rare disease that Dr. Chen didn't call cancer, even though it acts like cancer with uncontrollable growth of the neoplasms. Unlike cancer, however, LAMN does not spread to other parts of the body through the blood or the lymph system. The problem would be contained in my abdominal cavity. The good news was I didn't have ovarian cancer, and also that the LAMN were slow growing, giving us time to figure out my next steps.

I finally had a diagnosis, but it came with the conditional message that we were waiting for the completion of the pathology report for further information on how to proceed. Either I was heavily drugged or those speaking to me were terribly unclear, but I didn't end up with a good understanding of what these results all meant. I was relieved to hear that I didn't have ovarian cancer. Those who spoke to me were emphasizing that positive news, but I felt an undercurrent of something much darker behind their words. In my confusion, I remember a physician assistant making eye contact with me and saying, "The most important thing right now is to focus on recovering from this surgery. Then you'll be ready to deal with whatever comes further down the road." That made the most sense of anything anyone had said to me.

I left the hospital the day after my surgery and was told I would be referred to a doctor in their gastrointestinal surgical oncology program for follow up.

Eli was waiting outside the hospital door to pick me up. I learned that he had been kept informed of my situation. I was still quite confused about it all and happy to hear him recount what the doctor had told him. We began our long drive home. It wasn't just Eli who had come forward with his support. Another one of my sons, Gabriel, had offered to drive down from his home in Washington state and stay with me for a week while I recovered. As Eli drove me home, we learned that Gabe had been able to drive further than he'd anticipated and would be waiting for us at my house when we got there.

As a district park ranger in North Cascades National Park, Gabe's workload was lighter at the time, but things were about to ramp up for Spring. Still, he felt he could take the time away. His wife Stacy, a physical therapist, had help from her mom living nearby to care for their two young children. They worked out the childcare, and so Gabe could come to help me. I thanked Stacy profusely. She is a "can-do" person and responded, "Of course we want to help. Gabe was there for me when my parents had their car accident. I'm glad he can come to you and help." Still, I knew I was causing disruption in their family, and I was concerned about that.

All three of my sons had been extremely independent from early on in their adult lives. I knew they loved me, but I was a bit taken aback by their ready offers to help. I too am extremely independent and not great at asking for or accepting help in general, but I felt so vulnerable as I wandered in the darkness of all this surprising health news. I hadn't had surgery since my tonsils were removed when I was four. I wasn't sure what I would need in this new chapter. In the end, I accepted the help offered by my sons. As Eli drove me home, I was already coming to understand how much their help meant to me. I couldn't have felt more supported, more loved. I was so very grateful.

Chapter 2

Stumbling Into the Big Picture

I followed the advice of the physician's assistant and went home to heal from the surgery. I didn't like hearing that I was being referred to a gastrointestinal oncological surgeon. I particularly didn't like hearing the surgeon part. *Wouldn't that mean there was more surgery in my future?* I hoped not. My mom was famous for offering up old sayings at times like this. It used to annoy me no end, but now that she is gone, I come up with these things myself. Often, they actually help. What wafted through my mind then was, *Only time will tell,* and with that, I was able to put these thoughts in the background of my life rather than keeping them right up front. As I waited to hear from the new doctor, it was enough to concentrate on my healing.

I was careful to follow the doctor's instructions about my physical recovery, but I also wanted to look within for inner guidance as I navigated this new terrain. I turned to my tried-and-true ways for communing with my deeper self: making art and paying attention to my dreams.

I am not trained as an artist. In fact for most of my life I was certain that I couldn't draw anything at all. I was lost in our society's trance about making art. That trance leads us all to believe that only the gifted few are allowed to be artists, leaving most of the rest of us shuddering with shame when asked to draw something. Children are allowed to express themselves freely in the arts, but it is disheartening how early we lose that sense of free expression, how soon we decide we aren't "good enough." Most have given it up completely by early adolescence if not before. We set aside a huge part of our basic humanity when we leave making art behind. We become spectators instead of participants and only vaguely realize what we might be missing.

It wasn't until I was in my forties that I opened the door to my own artmaking. I came to my creative life through music, returning to playing the piano in mid-life. I was interested in exploring music therapy when I started my master's degree program in psychology, but my mentor was an art therapist. She helped me open the door to making art. It was from her that I learned to let go of what my art looked like and ask rather what my art was trying to tell me. It turned out that my art had a lot to say, that it reached beneath the stories I was telling myself about what I thought or felt and helped me discover non-verbally more about what was really going on inside of me.

Most importantly, making art and playing music as an adult helped me open to the vast world of my imagination and all the gifts that come from that magical part of being human. A paucity of imagination leads to a habitual, drab existence. An active, alive imagination is life-giving, and opens our eyes to a world of new possibilities. Opening to making art and enlivening my imagination awakened me to the reality of my inner life and offered a way to communicate with this non-verbal part of myself.

Communicating Through Art and Dreams

When I turned to art after my surgery, I was basically reflecting inwardly with these thoughts and questions: *What has happened to me? How am I holding this experience inside? What meaning am I to take from it all?* I held those thoughts loosely in my mind and turned to my imagination to see what it wanted to tell me. Making art, for me, is a dance between my unconscious mind and my conscious mind. I try to let the unconscious part of me lead, and I ask my conscious mind to follow.

I focused on the empty space in my abdomen that was once home to the part of me that made the miracle of birth possible. For me, at 75, a hysterectomy is not a tragedy. As my son Gabriel said to the doctor, "Those parts did their job. They served me very well." "Yes," I said, picking up on his humor. "Look what they produced," and proudly pointed to my three sons on the screen, where they were joining my appointment remotely that day.

I rarely know what I'm going to paint before I see it appear on the paper. Here, I knew only that I wanted to paint something about the terrain of my abdomen minus all that had been removed. What emerged was the peace of the universal night with a full moon shining brightly in that now empty space, a picture I titled *Emptiness and the Night Sky*.

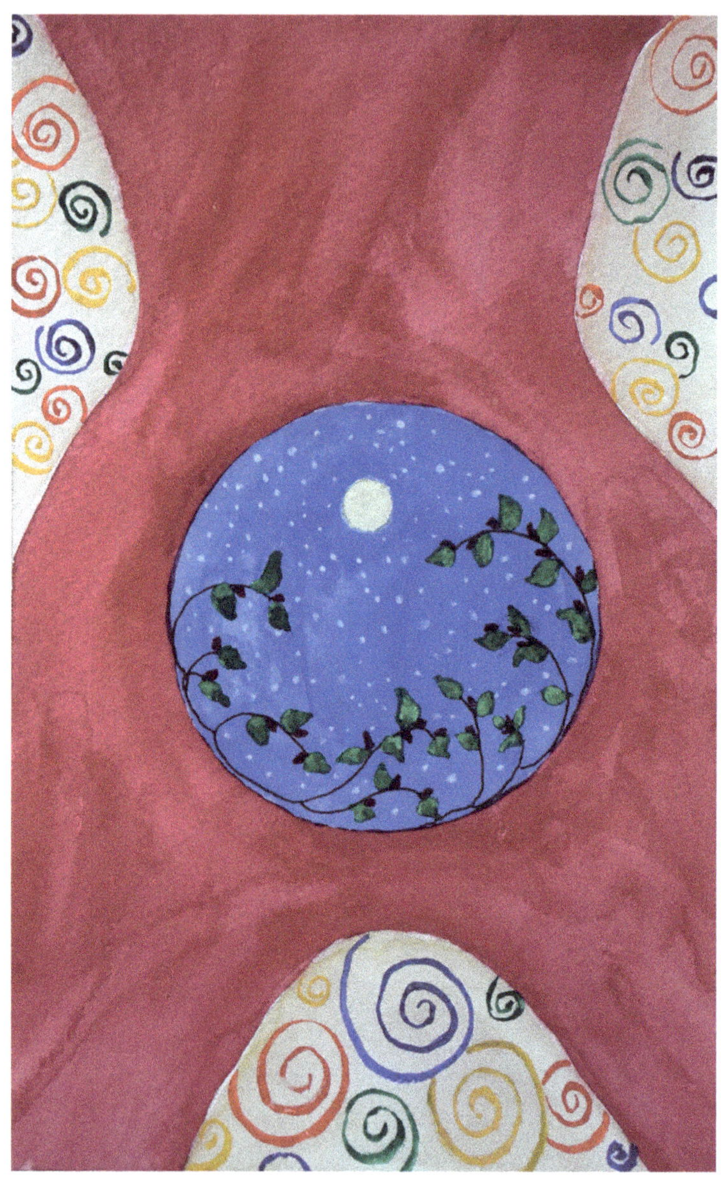

Emptiness and the Night Sky

I hold the moon and its reflective light as a deeply feminine image. In spite of the loss of those organs so essential to
my womanhood, when I looked at what I had created, I was

comforted to find my undisturbed connection to the universal energy of the deep feminine. The mystery of the night sky gave me a large enough perspective to hold the multiplicity of feelings I was experiencing as I waited to hear what would happen next. This piece of art did help me to reorient after my surgery. It helped me to find the balance I needed to move forward.

My dreams are another way I have learned to communicate with my unconscious mind. I have been recording and working with my dreams since my twenties. Our dreams are one of the things that convinces me that we humans are all creative in our very core. We make up the most impossible stories, complete with moving pictures, and tell them to ourselves every night. We don't, however, always remember them, but we can all cultivate a relationship with this part of ourselves and learn how dreams communicate with us through body energy, image, symbol, and story. They have always felt to me like a direct communication from my soul. I knew they would be helpful to me in my healing journey.

Looking to my dreams for guidance after my surgery was a bit more challenging than usual because I had some trouble remembering them. I blamed that on the anesthesia, but I don't know if that was true. When I did remember, my dreams were compact, more often a single image rather than a story. One of those images was particularly impactful. It spoke loudly about the ultimate materiality of our human existence, a sobering fact that in this circumstance I found hilariously funny on waking.

Dreams often pick up fragments of our waking life experiences and use them as fodder to communicate deeper meaning in the dream world. This dream looked to my garbage as a metaphor to deliver its message. I live in the country. To reduce odors and discourage the raccoons, foxes and yes, even bears, from making a terrible mess of my refuse, I freeze all my food waste in a bag and put it in my garbage can, frozen, on pickup day. My dream world surprised me by using this part of my day world to communicate an important message to me.

Here is my dream as I wrote it in my journal that morning:

I am a bag of frozen compost! I am in two places at once, both inside and outside of this image. I can feel what it is like to be the compost, but I can also see the mishmash of colors in the bag from the outside, the orange of citrus peels, the green of kale stems, the brown of onion skins, etc. As I rise out of a deep sleep toward waking, I feel/see the bag beginning to defrost with all the frozen pieces coming apart.

I opened my eyes with a startle. My dream had taken place as I crossed the bridge from sleep to waking. This made waking up feel like a movie with visuals, movement, and a felt sense. I often marvel at the brilliance of the imagination and its ability to present a complex, deeply felt truth in a single image. This dream was a perfect example of that, as despite everything we humans think we are, on the material plane, we are in the end, compost! While I might have had a more somber reflection at another time, awakening in the vitality of my dream, I could only laugh—not just a giggle, but a big deep belly laugh. I titled this dream, *My Awakening*.

Dreams and art come from the same place inside of us. Bringing them together in the waking world, doubles their power to communicate. They work in tandem. I often paint my dream images. My paintings bring something new forward that a future dream picks up on. Sometimes synchronicities from my waking life join in with related content and the circle goes round and round. It becomes like imaginary play. I can't wait to see what is going to happen next.

A Collage Series Brings Deeper Understanding

I immediately felt called to do some art about my bag of compost dream. In a gut level decision, I decided to make a colored paper collage. Unbeknownst to me at the time, I ended up doing a series of paper collages that lived my dream forward to an important insight.

The first one, *Frozen Compost Marilyn*, is of me pictured under the night sky.

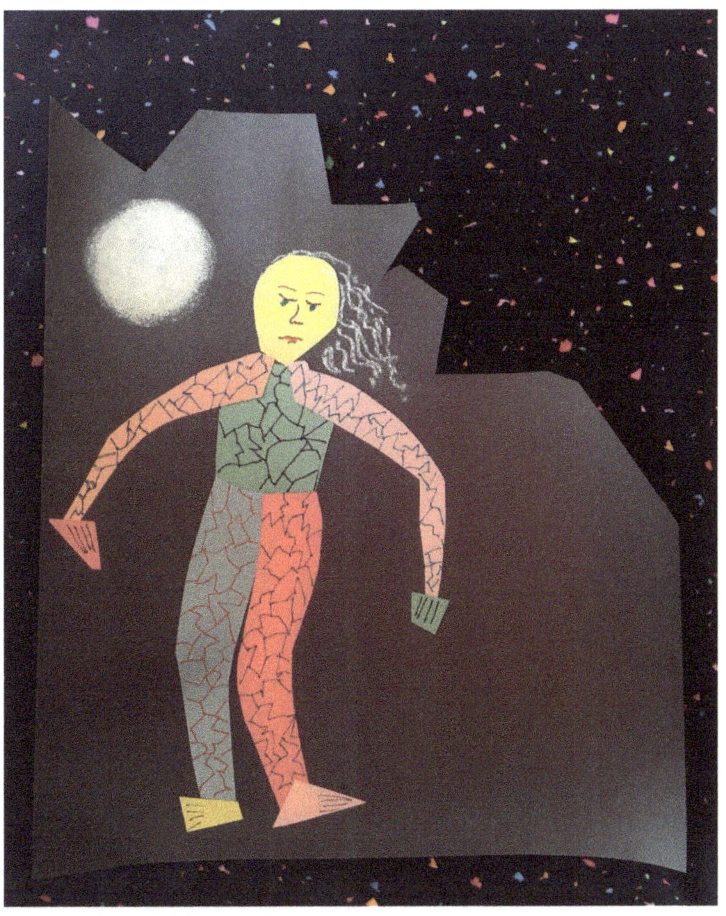

Frozen Compost Marilyn

It expresses how I felt as the frozen bag of compost. I immediately noticed that it looked like a puzzle. The puzzle, which is me, is made up of many different parts, but they all work together to hold shape and form, as me. When I imagined myself there in that shape, I felt my stiffness, a bit like the Tin Man in the Wizard of Oz.

As I felt the stiffness, I was anxious to express myself thawing, so I made another collage. *Melting Compost Marilyn* shows me pictured under the moon and the sun.

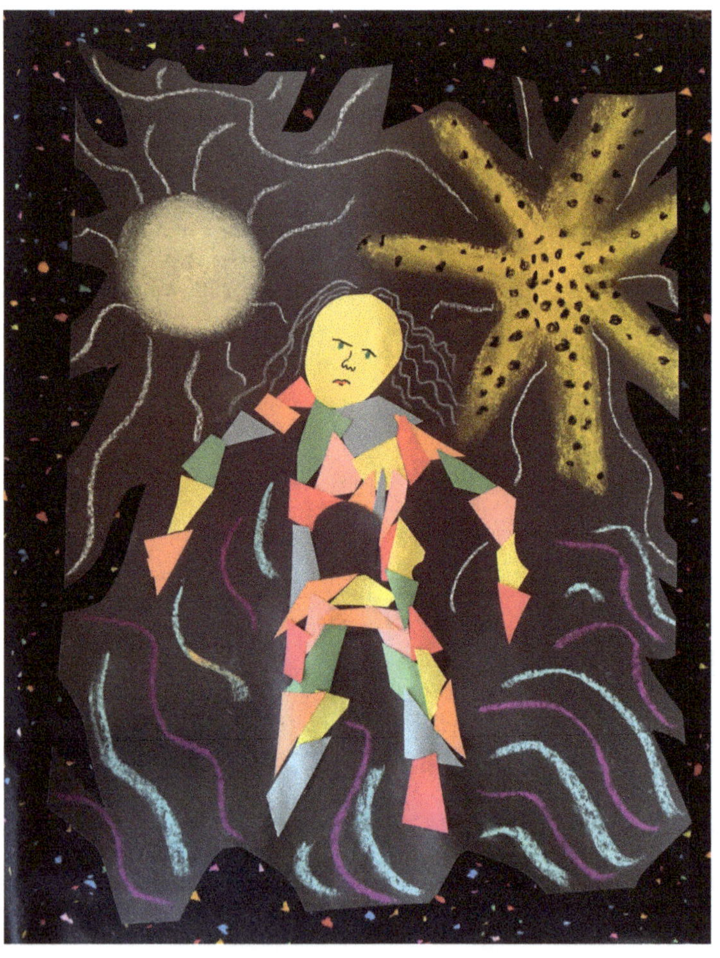

Melting Compost Marilyn

On my dawn walks, I marvel on those days when the full moon lays itself down into the ocean in the West, just as the sun is rising in the East. To me, that is a magical time when day and night exist as one. Thinking symbolically, I was reminded by my collage that the rational me (Sun Marilyn) and the non-rational me (Moon Marilyn) can access the wisdom of each of these spheres. When those energies find balance with one another, there is movement, things are shaken up, and with that loosening more things seem possible.

In this collage, I saw that the colors had shattered and were mixing as energy moves in my body. The blank space of my hysterectomy was framed by the movement, now a mysterious inner space, still healing and not yet ready to be filled with something new. As I pasted the shattered pieces, I could feel the movement, the freedom, and the possibility embodied here. My art was taking on a life of its own and dreaming my dream forward.

As I allowed myself to surrender to that much disintegration, I became deeply concerned about whether my form would hold. *Could I handle that much breaking apart?* I wondered. I left my art pieces out on the table so I could walk by them each day. I was wondering if more wanted to be expressed and waited for further inspiration. A friend who looked at my art suggested I enter my imagination and play with that edge where so much movement left me concerned about my form holding. Experimenting, I was able to let the movement increase, exaggerating it even, and what I found was even more freedom and vitality. I wanted to express that and made another collage.

When I began working on this next piece, the only thing I knew was that the colors needed to be circles. I found my hole punch and set to work. As I was finishing, I decided to put the old angular shards around the edges. When I stepped back and looked, I saw them as falling away, being pushed out by the new energy of the circles.

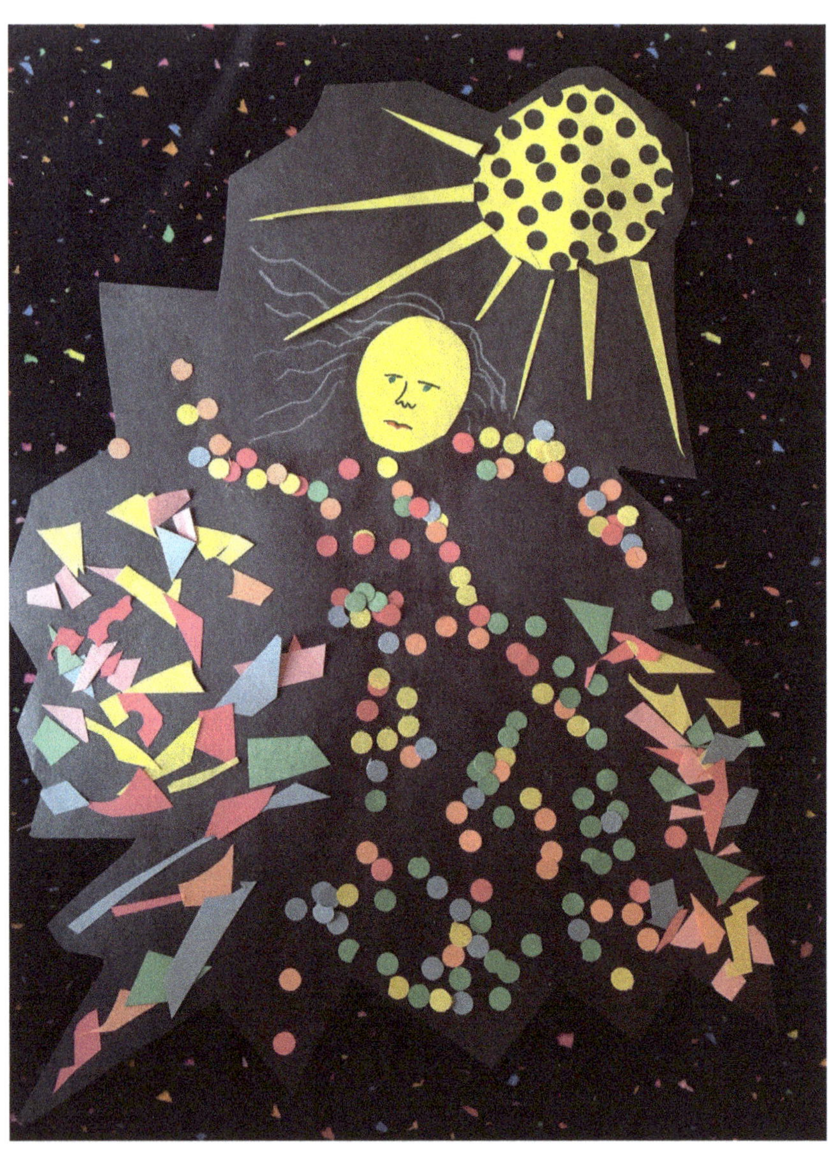

Transforming Marilyn

I am only partly recognizable here, certainly a far cry from *Frozen Compost Marilyn*. This collage brought thoughts of metamorphosis. If it were possible to depict what happens in the cocoon as a caterpillar turns into butterfly, this, I imagined, is what it might look like. I titled this collage *Transforming Marilyn*. She dances under a spotted sun.

I was puzzled for some time about why I felt called to cut away at the black background in my collages. I had no memory of doing that before in my art, though I may have. As I sat with my three pieces, it came to me that perhaps I was expressing how I felt my future was being whittled away by my health crisis. I shared this with a friend, who, not liking that thought, told me she saw it as carving away my past rather than my future. *Hmm . . . something to consider,* I thought.

Another friend offered that my experience was bringing things down to what is essential. I liked that thought, too. How grateful I am to have friends who widen my perspective so! Sharing art and dreams with loved ones and asking for a response as if it were their dream or their art, is always enlightening. What I came to for myself was this thought: *if I am letting go of my past and feel my future being carved away, what is essential in my life right now might become more obvious. Certainly, the present moment, a place I struggle to live from, might not be quite as illusive.*

As I lived with my collages, I noticed how my head remained a constant element in each one. My gut began telling me that I needed to let my head go. That was disturbing because my head holds all the stories about who I think I am, all the patterns that make me, me. More than anywhere else in my body, my head is where my ego resides. If my goal was to surrender to the transformation that was trying to take place inside me, my head had to go, but it took me a while to gather the courage to make my next collage.

When I finally did it, I was amazed at the deep wisdom that emerged. I started this fourth collage by tipping my yellow head sideways on an empty sheet of black paper. Now, falling like Humpy Dumpty off the wall, my head was revealed to have an egg shape. Quickly, as I glued, the nest and the tree formed around the egg. The tree spilling itself down from the sky world made a bridge between heaven and earth, above and below. The energy that was my body was now part of the tree. I recognized that tree as the mythical *Tree of Life* and so gave that as the title to my collage.

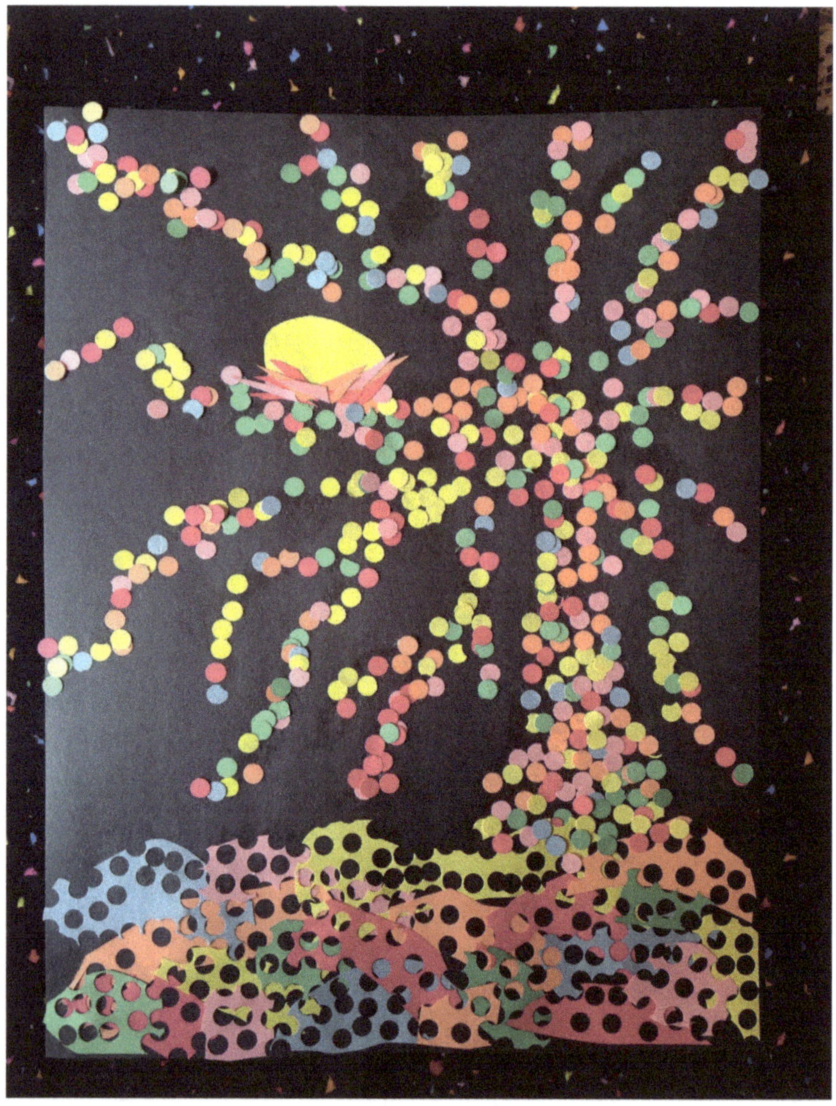

The Tree of Life

I had unconsciously created an image of the *axis mundi*; a mythical place imagined the world over as the center of it all. The place where everything begins and where everything ends in the never-ending circle of life. No one is excluded from that circle, and in it, we find our deepest belonging.

My collages were not planned by my conscious mind but fell onto the paper from a deeper place inside of me. I wasn't yet sure how serious my illness was, but I was being confronted with my mortality. The process of making my collages had led me, step by step, back to an awareness of the circle of life and reminded me that endings complete the circle out of which the new is constantly being born. I wanted to hold my life as part of that circle. My intuition had urged me to let my head fall, as only then could I come to a new understanding of the deeper truth about this moment in my life.

Placing my little life with all its earthly concerns in this larger perspective of the Tree of Life brought a deep sigh of relief. As when on my stormy walk on Christmas morning or finding the night sky where my uterus had been in my last painting, I could feel my surrender to the larger forces in which my life is held. Navigating the rough seas of my surgery and diagnosis, I had found again a place of peace in the eye of the storm. These moments were sustaining me through troubled times.

In my first book, *Finding the Wild Inside*, I tell the story of how I came to embrace my belonging in the circle of life, how that necessitated understanding that life's endings are absolutely as important as life's beginnings. My years caring for my elderly parents left me reflecting on death and dying, my own included. But at that time, I hadn't yet bumped up against something that fully awakened my own mortality from its partial slumber in the background of my life. Now, my health crisis was doing just that.

My four collages helped me return to thoughts about the circle of life. If asked, I would have related all that to my spiritual perspective on death and dying, but like many of our spiritual perspectives, I wasn't currently living from inside of that circle. Fearing for my life, I had become obsessed with the question of how much longer I might have to live. In my tunnel vision, I had unconsciously switched from feeling held in that circle to seeing my life in a linear fashion. When I looked at my lifeline, rather than seeing it stretching into a misty, undefined future, my illness had partially erased the line. It now ended in my clear view, closer to where I was standing.

The renowned mythologist, storyteller, and author Michael Meade, who often provides me with new insights, notes that we struggle with time, the loss of it or the lack of it, because what we long for is a connection to things outside of time, the eternal truths at the heart of our human existence. My collages, ending in the *Tree of Life*, had transported me to one of those "eternal truths."

The Path Forward

My personal health predicament continued to be mirrored in our larger world as the pandemic marched on. In my life as a patient, everything had been tossed up in the air, and I wasn't at all sure how things would come down again. I had been forced from my comfortable routines and expected outcomes into a time of deep unknowing. Because of the pandemic, the same thing was happening to all those around me. The world was in chaos and so was my life. The truth is none of us knows what is going to happen from one moment to the next. As much as I don't like it, I know there is power in uncertainty. It brings us closer to the life/death/life door where some things need to pass away, and other things need to be born. If I was looking for change, I had found my way to a propitious place.

While I hoped I was not going to die soon, I didn't want to come through this health crisis exactly as I was before I entered it. I wanted it to change me, to take me to a more expansive version of myself. I know with everything in me that creation comes out of chaos. If I wanted change, rather than me nibbling around the edges of stability to bring it about, radical change was more likely to manifest when my old patterns were shattered. My illness had certainly dealt a blow to my old patterns, and my collages were giving me a detailed picture of that process.

To make the change you want to happen, I was learning, you can't hold on to a frozen notion of who you think you are or how you think things should be. Better to open to the creative power deep inside and listen to your instincts and intuitions about what is trying to emerge. In the heat of the creative fire, there is no going back to normalcy. Having entered into the process of metamorphosis, who among us would want to emerge from the cocoon as a caterpillar rather than a butterfly?

My frozen compost dream marked a path forward for me, a path on which I hoped to walk as an ever-changing Marilyn, authentically following my heart and my dreams to my last days. In that way, no matter how much time I had left on this earth, I would find my way to a life fully lived. That was what I most hope for.

Chapter 3

Walking in the Weeds

The moments of peace I was finding in the midst of the storm were deeply nourishing and restorative. I felt buoyed by this big perspective on what I was living through, but as is true in life, I wasn't able to stay with those big thoughts all the time. As time passed, dark clouds descended once again as I waited to hear from the UCSF surgeon's office. I was increasingly fearful about what might have to happen next.

In hopes of getting a better picture of what I was dealing with, I had read about my disease, LAMN (*low grade appendiceal mucinous neoplasms*) on the internet. I had poured over pathology reports, researching medical terminology that I didn't understand to try to determine the extent of my illness. It seemed my prognosis rested on the extent of my disease.

The nurse practitioner from Dr. Mohamed Abdelgadir Adam's office reached out to me in the middle of March, about a month after my hysterectomy. Fearing more surgery, the first question I asked was why I had been referred to a surgeon. She explained that Dr. Adam was a specialist in Appendiceal Cancer.

It was jarring to hear that word *cancer*. I had been comforting myself with Dr. Chen's words that LAMN was not cancer but acted like cancer. While I know it is not always true, somewhere inside me the cancer word came with a death sentence. I didn't want it anywhere near me. It turned out to be the last time my disease would be described that way at UCSF, but I didn't know that at the time.

The nurse practitioner affirmed that "low grade" meant the neoplasms were slow growing so there wasn't a rush for treatment. She ordered blood tests and told me I would need to have a CT scan before I saw the doctor. When I asked about the severity of my disease, her response was, "I think I'll let Dr. Adam answer that question. He has such a good way of talking about it." I confessed to her that while waiting to hear from their office, I 'd been reading about my diagnosis on the internet. Trying to be encouraging, I think, she said, "You have probably read about the CRS/HIPEC treatment then, yes?" I hadn't. She gave me a link.

When we finished our phone call, I sat down with my laptop and typed in the link she had given me. There I found lovely testimonials from people who had gone through the treatment, followed by an animated video about the procedure itself. I clicked the little arrow and watched with horror as a narrator calmly described what was happening in the video. First, they made an incision from the sternum to the pelvis, so the abdomen was fully open. Next, they carefully searched for and removed all of the visible offending neoplasms. The patient was temporarily sewed back together in preparation for the chemotherapy bath. Hoses then delivered hot chemotherapy to the closed abdomen. The patient's belly was massaged for 90 minutes in order to move the chemo into every possible nook and cranny of the abdomen. After that, they rinsed the chemo from the abdomen and stitched the patient up for good.

Yikes! The surgery would likely be 6-8 hours long. The patient could expect to recover in the hospital for weeks. To me, that alone indicated the seriousness of the operation, as in this day and age, barely functioning patients are usually rushed out the hospital door with great haste.

When the video was over, I could hardly breathe. This was never going to happen to me, of that, I was sure. It didn't seem even vaguely in the realm of possibility for a 75-year-old woman like me. I simply couldn't imagine it. As I shut down my computer, I hoped with all my heart that there was some other way to deal with my condition.

Dreaming A New Perspective

Soon after, I recalled a dream I'd had a couple of weeks earlier. I had done a painting about the dream at the time and that image kept flashing in my mind. I looked back in my journal so I could reread the dream and recall all the details. At the time I'd had the dream, I felt it was speaking to the surprise of my medical situation, but in revisiting my dream and my artwork, a deeper message was revealed. This was my dream:

I am in a small room at an airport. I can see through a window that there is an airplane parked too close to the terminal. When the plane starts moving, I leap up from where I am sitting and run to the back of the room. Had I stayed where I was, I would have been crushed because the wall has crumbled, and the plane has entered that corner of the building. Standing there by the exit door, I survey the damage. It is as if the plane is turned inside out, and what is protruding through the wall is not the outer nose of the plane but rather a huge black metal instrument panel with blinking orange and red lights.

The black metal instrument panel was the part of the dream that I then painted.

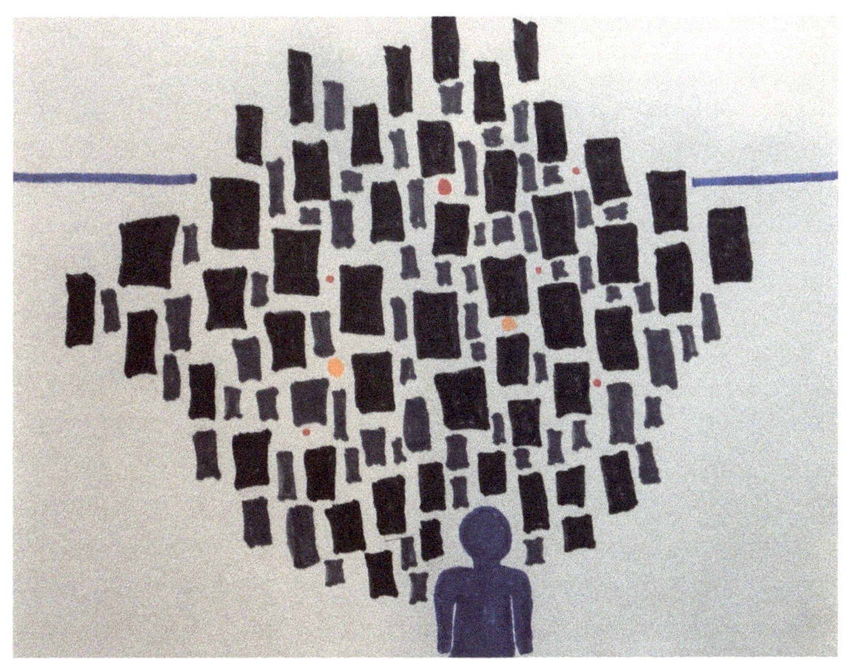

The Pilot's Perspective Revealed

Upon waking, the nightmarish quality of the dream left me with a strong experience of what it is like to be confronted by something completely unexpected. It reminded me of how my diagnosis had burst into my reality with such great surprise to healthy Marilyn, catapulting me into this new world of being a patient. Now the frightening video about the CRS/HIPEC treatment had burst through the wall of my consciousness like the airplane bursting through the wall in my dream. It confronted me with a treatment that was so frightening it seemed completely impossible to endure.

My dream had commented on what I already knew about my medical situation, but I wanted to see if it had information about how to deal with it all. When I relived the dream in my mind, I saw the airplane parked too close to the terminal and heard the setting of my dream as "the terminal" addressing whether my ill health was a terminal situation. I saw myself flee from my original seat where I certainly would have been crushed by this event. That made me feel like there was something I could do to help save myself. Then I saw the wall start to crumble and the big black piece of metal resembling a control panel enter the room. The bumbling airplane was terrifying when I saw it from the outside moving too close to the building, but when it turned inside out, my dream offered me the whole new reality, that of the pilot's perspective in the cockpit.

My world looked completely different when sitting in the pilot's seat. I was in control. No longer dominated by the overwhelming size of the threat I perceived from the outside, I simply had to step into the pilot's seat and from moment to moment respond to whatever arose. Now each of those little black rectangles in my drawing, seemed to represent moments in time, each of them viewed from the pilot's position, manageable. I knew that having this dream didn't solve my problem, but it was pointing me in the right direction.

First Meeting with Dr. Adam

It was April Fool's Day when I finally met with Dr. Adam at the Mission Bay campus of UCSF. Nothing about that day seemed funny to me. If there were tricks and pranks being played, it seemed like they were being played on me by the gremlin of ill health. I desperately needed more information about what I was dealing with, but I was terrified to hear what he might have to say.

My dear friend Joanna had driven me from Mendocino to UCSF but could not come into my appointment because of the pandemic. All three of my sons were able to attend my appointment virtually that day. I felt so well supported by all their loving energy and their willingness to help see me through this challenge.

When Dr. Adam came into the room, I was so nervous, I wanted to jump out of my skin. We were both masked, which left us both partially hidden. I was happy to be hiding, but his mask made it harder for me to receive the cues I depended on to determine if he was friend or foe. My glasses were fogging with each breath, and I kept removing them. I was trying desperately to sense something about who this man was.

Was he someone I could trust?

I noticed right away that he seemed very confident but was not overly full of ego. His presence left plenty of space for me in the room. If there was distance between us, it was coming from me, not him. My fear left me struggling to be open as he explained more about my diagnosis of LAMN.

"Calling what you have cancer is somewhat controversial," he said. "I prefer not to because the neoplasms are benign tumors, and we don't treat them by using systemic chemotherapy. What you have is a surgical disease. LAMN does need to be treated . . ." He paused and with an edge of regret in his voice that maybe I only imagined, he finished his sentence. ". . . And even after we surgically remove the neoplasms, they tend to come back."

I was happy about distancing myself from the C-word, but I didn't like hearing that last part. As we talked, I was able to let my guard down and become more receptive as we went on. "The good news is that the neoplasms do not penetrate the abdominal wall," he continued, "and they do not spread to other parts of the body through the blood or the lymph system." His voice was calm and reassuring, but I was on a roller coaster ride, my hope rising when what he said was positive and crashing down when what he said frightened me.

We asked a lot of questions. *Do they know what causes my disease? How long did he think the neoplasms had been growing in my abdomen? Why didn't I have symptoms?* There wasn't a single moment when I felt rushed, not a single hint that he needed to move on to his next patient. He remained completely present in the room with us and patiently responded to each inquiry.

"The cause of LAMN is unknown, and the neoplasms were probably growing there for a couple of years. Some people do have symptoms, but most are diagnosed in a roundabout way like you were, a surgery for something else, and then the neoplasms are discovered." He then described the treatment.

"The CRS/HIPEC procedure is the treatment for LAMN. It is a very aggressive procedure," he admitted, emphasizing the word *aggressive*, or maybe I just heard it that way. From the way he spoke, I understood that he meant it was the only treatment. He briefly explained what the procedure involved. I shivered as I recalled that video.

When he finished, I asked, "At the end of the scary video I watched on the internet, it was mentioned that doctors are trying to figure out how to do this surgery laparoscopically. Might that be possible for me?" My thought was that not having to have my whole abdomen cut open might help me imagine this treatment as a possible choice.

"That is a bit disingenuous," he replied, "because it isn't usually the incision that causes the problems." I don't think he knew he was dashing my only hope. I was too overwhelmed at that point to ask what did cause the problems if not the incision, or maybe I just didn't want to know.

Dr. Adam paused to see how I was responding. Perhaps he sensed my fear because he then said, "This really isn't such a bad diagnosis, you know." The room was silent while I tried to let his words into my reality. I realized he was probably used to dealing with devastating disease, and that he might see my situation as not as bad as some, but in that moment, I couldn't really find the place inside me that agreed.

The appointment progressed, and I learned that my blood tests were back in the normal range after my hysterectomy and the CT scan was not ringing any alarm bells. He asked if he could examine my abdomen. His hand was warm and gentle as he pressed all around, asking me if anything was uncomfortable. He commented to his assistant that my belly was soft.

I gathered that this was a good thing. "We will be monitoring you regularly for changes," he said, completing the exam. I didn't need to take further action at this time but could think about all we had talked about. He would see me again in three months.

At the very end of my appointment. Dr. Adam looked at me and said, "You seem very lucid." That stopped me in my tracks. *Lucid*? No one had yet commented on my lucidity or lack of it—I thought that it was assumed I was alert and clear mentally. Sitting there worried and masked, I wondered if I looked especially old that day, giving him cause to project a stereotype. Teasing him, I replied, "I think maybe I'm experiencing ageism at UCSF." We both laughed. He apologized and said it was just my age demographic, that at 75 I was in better shape than many people he sees. Looking back, perhaps he was beginning to evaluate whether I might be a candidate for surgery, but I wasn't considering that at the time.

My sons laughed when we talked about that comment after my appointment. Eli's take on it was that maybe Dr. Adam thought my sons were attending because I wasn't mentally competent. It strikes me very funny now, but in the moment, I felt really old, like the first time I was asked if I qualified for a senior discount. This first comment on my lucidity suggested maybe I had now entered old, old age, and since my age was my biggest concern in regard to treating my disease, I was unsettled. Still, I liked Dr. Adam right from the start. He seemed like someone I could trust.

I was relieved that nothing needed to happen immediately. April had brought springtime energy. When I felt like I had healed physically from my hysterectomy, I set out on a solo road trip to visit my sons and their families. I'd gotten my second Covid shot and was raring to go. Because of the pandemic, I hadn't seen my little grandsons in more than a year. My relationship with the littlest boys consisted of my reading them stories on Zoom. The older boys didn't love Zoom, so I'd been writing them letters.

I made a big circle from my coastal California home in Mendocino to Utah, to the state of Washington, then back down the California coast to home. While I had downloaded audiobooks for my journey, I had trouble concentrating and preferred to just let my mind wander as I drove for miles and miles under big open skies of the American West. I wanted to leave all my health concerns behind and start fresh with what was most important to me, my family. I returned home in early May with a clear mind and a warm heart, ready to pick up my life and move forward.

Before I knew it, summer was upon us. On the Mendocino Coast the months of June and July bring coastal fog as temperatures rise inland. My morning walks were damp and enshrouded in a mist that left nothing clearly defined. It seemed my mood and my thinking had become a little foggy as well.

My next appointment with Dr. Adam was scheduled for the middle of July. As the appointment neared, I became increasingly uneasy. It began to dawn on me that there were next steps, and perhaps now I was going to have to take them. Either that or be grateful for the life I've lived and surrender to my disease. I had asked Dr. Adam how I would die if I died from LAMN. He thought probably from a bowel obstruction. That didn't sound good at all, but I was still not thinking of the CRS/HIPEC procedure he'd described as even a remote possibility for me.

Lessons from Labyrinth Walks

When I'm feeling off balance or in a quandary, I have a meditative practice of walking the labyrinth. I had constructed one in a meadow on my land a few years back. In the week before my next appointment with Dr. Adam, an enormous tension was building inside me, so I turned to walking the labyrinth to try to bring some focus and peace. In one day, I walked two different labyrinths. What happened in both surprised me.

The labyrinth is an ancient pattern dating back some 5000 years. It is based on the spirals and circles found in nature and has been found in cultures the world over. It is not a maze. There are no tricks to it and no dead ends. It has a single circuitous path that winds its way to the center. Symbolically, as you walk this path, you find your way to your own center. Exiting the same way you entered, you leave in closer touch with a deeper part of yourself as you step back into life's challenges.

A friend of mine had made a labyrinth on her property, and the lines marking the path were made up of different kinds of flowering bulbs. In March, first the daffodils bloomed, and by April the tulips arrived. These were followed a bit later by the irises. I hadn't been to her labyrinth since the tulips were in full bloom but figured by now, mid-summer, the irises had bloomed and faded. My visit was prompted by a friend who loves labyrinths coming to visit me in early July. She wanted to see the flower labyrinth, even though I told her the flowers would be long gone. I called my friend who had the labyrinth, and off we went to her house. The labyrinth was situated in her peaceful garden at the edge of the forest. I missed the wild display of color that had been there before, but we decided to walk the labyrinth anyway.

The shadows were lengthening in the late afternoon when I set out down the circular path. I was enjoying the light at that time of day and the dancing shadows cast by the breeze in the pine trees at the perimeter of the garden. The labyrinth path itself was covered with wood chips that crunched beneath my feet with each step I took. The area where the beautiful bulbs had blossomed was now in disarray, full of spent bulbs and beginning to be overtaken by weeds.

As is my practice when I am walking the labyrinth, I try to remain open to whatever presents itself, so as I walked amidst the disarray, I was thinking about chaos. Soon my mind was busy with thoughts: *I should come over and help my friend weed this. Maybe I should just pull a few of these weeds as*

I walk. I recalled the beauty of the flowers on my earlier visits and reflected with sadness on their passing. Even with that rotation of the bulbs, the blooms can't last forever. *Life doesn't last forever,* was my next thought. *Yes, my life can't last forever.* It seemed a time to contemplate that thought, which is what I did for the remainder of my meditative walk to the center of the labyrinth.

It was getting late when reluctantly I stepped out of the center and began to circle my way back to the path's exit. Now the chaotic landscape matched exactly how I felt inside. As I walked, I remembered my life before all my medical issues emerged. Back then, I was feeling the ripening of old age. My book, *Finding the Wild Inside,* had just come out the year before. There was a sense that I was in full bloom. Now suddenly, I was walking in the weeds.

There couldn't have been a clearer picture of how my life felt at that moment. I didn't want to be where I was. I wanted my health back, not this walk in the weeds, but the truth of this moment in my life was being presented to me, and I knew I needed to accept it. I began to repeat, *I am walking in the weeds. I am walking in the weeds,* like a mantra, letting the truth of it sink deeper inside me. *It is easier to accept the truth than expend energy trying to avoid it,* I thought to myself. I was charmed that a weed-ridden labyrinth would take me to the place of peace I found as I stepped off the path and back out into the garden.

Later that night, still amazed at what had been revealed earlier, I decided to go into my meadow and walk my own labyrinth before I went to bed. I live in the forest. It was a dark night. I had only enough light in the labyrinth to barely mark the path for night-time walking. Under a star-filled sky, I passed through the arch that marks the opening of the path and walked on towards the center. I felt the sureness in my footsteps, a steadiness in my body, and the exhilaration of being outdoors in the forest at night. It was so quiet. It was easy to open wide to the great mystery of life under the night sky with the living, breathing forest surrounding me.

When I reached the center of the labyrinth, I turned to face the little altar where I had placed tokens of the four elements—Earth, Fire, Water, and Air. I took a deep breath to settle myself in my center, but at that very moment, the silence was pierced by a wild bark. It was a sound I recognized as a fox and came from the bushes just a few feet away from me. I jumped, a scream escaping from my throat before I could stifle it. My heart was suddenly pounding. I wanted to run to my front door, but I stood frozen in place at the center of the labyrinth.

It flashed in my mind that something like this had happened before. I was in my hot tub enjoying the peace of the night when a fox barked loudly from the bushes behind me. I screamed and splashing water every which way, all six feet of me leaped out of the hot tub. Completely naked, I ran back into my house, sat down at my computer and Googled, Do foxes eat people? What I read assured me that, rabies aside, foxes don't often attack people, and if I felt threatened, it was more likely a fox was protecting its young.

As this memory flashed quickly through my mind, I yelled back to the fox. "Hey, what's up!" I waited but there was no response. "What are you doing out there?" I paused. I felt safer making sound than standing there paralyzed in the silence. "Are you protecting your babies?" I shouted into the night. No response, not a single sound emanated from the undergrowth at the base of those big redwood trees where I was sure the fox was hiding.

As I stood there wondering what to do, I became determined to finish my labyrinth walk. I stepped out of the center, now going along the path twice the speed I was going when I entered. Literally shaking, I sped down the path. Peering into the darkness, I was scanning the forest all around me, sometimes sensing energies from behind me, turning to face whatever it might be, shouting out when need be. My heart continued to pound.

At last, I exited the labyrinth, right by where I had heard the fox bark. I almost ran into the house, but as I approached the steps to my deck, a picture flashed in my mind's eye. I saw myself, as if from an aerial view, scurrying out of the labyrinth, and I burst out laughing. Anyone watching would have thought I'd gone mad. I had acted out of fear, fed by an active imagination and a sensitive heart. All this from one bark of a nearby fox who, for all I knew, might have just been trying to say hello and ask me what the heck I was doing, walking in circles in the meadow in the dark of the night!

I couldn't stop laughing when I got to safety, and I still have to laugh when I think about it. I had been tying myself in knots with fear about my upcoming appointment with Dr. Adam. My encounter with the fox, as I stood in the very center of the labyrinth, put me deeply in touch with myself, and who I was in that moment was fear personified! My experience loosened those knots I had tied and let the fear move freely through my body. It was physical, and it had found full expression.

So that is what fear looks like, I thought to myself as that aerial movie of my labyrinth walk played out in my mind again and again. *Fear spins itself into a tight ball in my mind, and this is what it really looks and feels like in my body.* All my shouting suddenly felt like my own version of barking. I had acted out the exact drama at the base of all my fear about my illness—*Will I survive this?*

I wrote extensively in *Finding the Wild Inside* about how my experiences in nature helped me through difficult times. Those stories were about elk, fish, and bears. Now the fox was coming to my aid. My encounter that night helped me hold my fear differently. I still wonder what the fox made of it all.

As the days ticked off and my appointment neared, I wasn't without fear, but the fear I felt remained grounded in my body, no longer that earlier sense of panic, spinning round and amplifying itself in my mind. Now, whenever I became aware of the fear, the hysterical laughter of my experience with the fox in the labyrinth came with it. I couldn't uncouple those two experiences, and the association made it feel a million times better. I felt ready to meet with Dr. Adam and hear what might happen next.

Chapter 4

Fear Bites

At my appointment in mid-July, I was surprised when Dr. Adam proposed a laparoscopic exploratory surgery to determine the extent of the disease in my abdomen. *Why didn't he mention that when I saw him before?* I thought in a panic. Would I have wanted to hear that so soon after my hysterectomy? I think not! Perhaps, like that nurse practitioner in the hospital, he was letting me heal from one surgery before he proposed the next. Now it had been five months since that surgery, but it still felt recent to me. It took me a minute to even consider what he was proposing. He assured me that my recovery would be much shorter than that previous surgery, but still I was hesitant.

"Really? Another surgery?" I said defensively. In a panic, I asked "Is it safe for me to go under anesthesia again so soon after my last surgery?"

He remained calm and assured me that it wasn't a problem. "You can think about it. There is no rush, but I recommend that we take this next step," he told me. "The CT scans only show so much, and by doing the exploratory surgery we will be much better informed about what we are dealing with."

50

While Dr. Adam was very relaxed and gave me permission to consider my situation, it was reassuring that he could also be very clear when there was something he thought needed to happen. I left my appointment with much to think about.

Gratitude for the Miracle of Healing

During the time I was mulling all this over, I awoke one morning from a dream that I felt was related to surgery. And I immediately wrote it down:

A young girl has been bitten by a fox. There are several lacerations on her body. I am wiping them to clean off caked blood. I am pressing hard, but it doesn't seem to be hurting her. She seems very thankful for the help.

I'm thinking about what the attack must have felt like when it was happening. As I am thinking this, I see three black and white snapshots of the fox biting her. It must have been really frightening for her when the attack happened, but she shows no sign of that fear now, nor does she speak about it. She was marked by it on her body. but she is moving forward.

Astonishingly, I was awakened abruptly from this dream by four loud barks from a fox who was sitting just outside my open bedroom window. Amazed by the synchronicity of the fox appearing in my waking life just as I was dreaming about a fox, I snuggled back down under my covers and tried to go back to sleep. I didn't succeed. I was shaken by the intensity of the dream and in awe that a real fox had come by as if to put an exclamation point on it.

Once again, a fox was playing a role in my healing journey. I have no explanation for why the fox barked and awakened me from my dream. When things like that happen, I experience the awe and wonder they bring in their wake, and then leave explanations to the mystery. But the fox barking had awakened me, and that meant I wasn't likely to forget my dream. Not only did I remember it, but my body was filled with the energy of the dream as I lay there in its aftermath. I had felt the trauma as I looked at those snapshots, and I had experienced the little girl's gratitude. The fox's bark delivered my dream across the bridge from sleep to my waking life.

I tossed and turned and thought about my dream. I realized that the girl's wound I was cleaning was just about the size of the tiny laparoscopic incisions made for my hysterectomy. Seeing the snapshots of the fox attacking, and my thought that it must have been a very frightening experience for her made me think about the surgery itself. We are anesthetized during surgery, so we won't feel pain or remember what went on, but I have often wondered what the body actually knows of the experience. The fact that the girl in my dream showed no sign of how frightening the experience was for her and doesn't speak about it, sounded a lot like the response of a person who has been anesthetized. Were the three black and white pictures of the fox attack telling me something about how frightening the surgery had been for the little girl who still lives inside of me? My mind was anesthetized, but I wondered, *Were the pictures telling me about the surgery from my body's perspective?*

I turned over onto my back and gave up trying to go back to sleep. Filled with the energy of the dream, both the terror and the gratitude, I instinctively found myself placing my hands on my abdomen as if I were trying to comfort the part of me that had experienced such trauma. I marveled that just these few months later, my body had completely healed. Suddenly, I was crying, not with sadness, but because I was literally overcome with gratitude for the healing power of the human body. This was not just a passing thought but a concrete experience of the innate power inside me, one that is inside all of us, to heal. It seemed nothing less than a miracle. I wept for some time until my tears subsided.

My dream had gifted me with everything I needed for this deeply felt healing moment to take place. Not only did I experience the miracle of our ability to heal, but also the miracle that our dreams are watching out for us, offering up in body energy and symbolic language important messages from our unconscious minds.

Back Down on Earth

Every year I look for that moment in late August when the angle of the light begins to shift, signaling that summer is coming to its end. I love the fall. Of all the changes in seasons, I cherish summer turning to fall the most. It was around this time I received a message from Dr. Adam's office that he wanted to schedule a virtual appointment with me. I wondered what that was about. Was there some new news? I was puzzled.

We met virtually in early September, and Dr. Adam didn't waste any time, telling me kindly but firmly that it was time to decide if I wanted to go ahead with the exploratory surgery. I find it hard to believe now, but I was surprised. In my mind, I thought I had months to think about it, but here we were only six weeks after it had been proposed.

I feel silly now as I should have known what was up. The fact that I didn't makes me realize the amount of denial I still had about my medical situation. My disease was floating there in my consciousness, but this conversation with Dr. Adam brought me back down to earth, back to the reality that I had an important decision to make.

Looking back, I had already made the choice. I just hadn't let myself realize it yet. In that appointment, when I told Dr.

Adam that I would go ahead with the surgery, I was hearing it for the first time myself. I can't help but think that my dream of the little girl and the fox, and the experience surrounding it helped me to make that decision and come to a peaceful resolve as I moved forward.

This time, my son Erik, oldest of the three, offered to come help me after the surgery. I argued mightily about his coming, as Dr. Adam had said this exploratory surgery would be so much easier to recover from than my hysterectomy. My friend Joanna had offered to drive me down and back from the surgery, but Erik insisted that he was going to come. He lives in Utah with his family and sells real estate in the Park City area. Having his own work schedule and ability to work remotely allowed him to come. He has two school-age sons, Andrew who was 11 at the time and Alex 8. Erik's wife Kristian, another can-do mom, supported Erik's coming, but again, I knew that an extra burden was being added to her load. I was sure I could be on my own when I returned home this time. I had been so grateful for the help of Gabe and Eli in my last surgery, but I was feeling badly about my needs messing with their families, as nice as all my daughters-in-law had been about it.

I had cared for my own parents in their later years. Now here I was being the parent who needed care. I really wanted to keep that to a minimum, but there was no stopping Erik. In the end, my friend Joanna drove me to UCSF to shorten Erik's drive from Utah. He arrived at the hospital in time to pick me up after my surgery.

Healing After Surgery

The surgery itself was uneventful. I was able to return home the same day. After the long drive, we came in the house, and I headed straight for my recliner in the living room. Erik sat down in the rocking recliner next to me. I remember looking over at him, my heart bursting with love as it always does when I am with my adult sons. As much as I hadn't wanted to disturb his life, I felt so taken care of. *What could be better for my healing?* I thought to myself. I decided to express my gratitude.

"Erik," I said, turning to look at him. "I realize maybe I could have managed this with friends. But after they brought me home and dropped me off, and then went on their way, I would have been sitting here all by myself. It probably would have been fine, but it's awfully nice to have you here with me. Thank you so much for coming."

Erik nodded. He had a look of satisfaction on his face that said, *I told you so.* It was clear to me that he sincerely wanted to come help me out. Erik was fifty-one. We had lived such independent lives for so long, and his life was incredibly busy. I'd been happy to look on from the periphery, but something switched inside me as we sat there. I got a double message from our conversation. I was more important to him than I consciously realized I was, and that, despite all his busyness, it was important to him to be a son who helps his mom in such a time as this.

At home, a couple of days after surgery, I stumbled upon something I didn't expect to find and couldn't explain away. I had been wearing the same dress since I returned from the hospital as it fell lightly over my abdomen and didn't press on my incisions. Driving home from the hospital, I had noticed that there was a dampness at my left shoulder. As I had been drinking while in a slightly reclined position in the hospital, I thought maybe it was just some water gone astray. My attention was focused on my abdomen not my shoulder, so it was another day or so before I realized that the wet spot on my dress was getting bigger and now was somewhat sticky.

Had I spilled food on my shoulder? How could that be? Now it had my attention. When I pulled the neck of my dress to the side, I realized that there was blood on my shoulder. The dark spot on my already dark green dress had grown increasingly larger over these couple of days. It was blood, and I was still bleeding.

I went in the bathroom, took off my dress and looked in the mirror. My upper arm was covered with caked blood. I couldn't see where it was coming from. I put my dress in the sink and ran cold water over it. Sure enough, the red blood dissolved in the water and turned the sink pink.

Where was this coming from? I found a washcloth and dampened it. I began wiping my upper arm carefully, but the blood was caked on there, and I had to press harder. It had been about a month since I'd had that dream about the little girl and the fox. I realized that I was now doing to myself exactly what I had done to the little girl in my dream. The smeared, caked blood looked exactly the same. I was making the identical motion, trying to find and then clean the wound. I couldn't help but see the connection. It brought the dream and the experience I'd had after waking into the present moment, just as I once again needed faith in my body's ability to heal. I had no explanation, but I was in awe at the synchronicity.

As I wiped, I eventually found a tiny cut, only about a quarter of an inch long there on outside of my upper arm. It must have been quite deep and only slowly seeping, or I would have noticed it sooner. I later found blood on the shoulder of the nightgown I had been sleeping in, as well. I was curious about what had caused this, but my major focus was on the amazement that my waking life had mirrored my dream.

I did email Dr. Adam's office to ask what might have caused the bleeding. To my surprise, Dr. Adam called me to learn more about it. He asked if I could send him a photo of the wound which I was happy to do. I joked with Erik that maybe someone had dropped a scalpel on me by mistake, but when I joked about that with Dr. Adam he was not laughing. He assured me that such an accident hadn't happened because he was there the whole time. I realized that he was taking this far more seriously than I was. The placement of the cut on the side of my upper arm made him think that a part of the operating table that presses in to assure stability of the patient during surgery may have been the cause of the problem. He apologized and told me that he would address this with his team, as he didn't want something like this to happen to another patient. I didn't ever hear what they found, but I was reassured by his concern.

Dr. Adam was responding to the physical problem that had presented itself while I was responding to the symbolic meaning of what had happened to me. I didn't try to tell him about my experience. I respected his time, and it was too long a story. I was grateful for his concern, but there was a part of me saddened that our two stories were destined to remain so separate. I was envisioning a world where the truth of both of our points of view could be held as one.

Chapter 5

A Turning Point

When I left the hospital after the exploratory surgery, Dr. Adam told me we would wait for the pathology report to determine my next step. As he had promised, my recovery was much quicker than when I'd had my hysterectomy.

When the report came back, it was time to make another pilgrimage down to UCSF for the results. Once again, my friend Joanna offered to go with me. The three-and-a-half-hour journey treated us to spectacular ocean views as we drove along the Pacific coast highway, and to the beauty of the redwood forest as we turned eastward to join more major highways. The vineyards through the wine country were showing signs of early fall on this last day in September. After living in the country for so long, it is always a bit jarring to join the freeway, cross the Golden Gate Bridge, and then cope with city traffic. I was grateful my friend was driving.

In my appointment, Dr. Adam told me that I still had options. He handed me a copy of the pathology report and scooted his chair next to me so we could go over the results together. We were both masked, but because of my habit of social distancing during

the pandemic, I was distracted by feeling a body so close to mine.
I don't know if I was concerned about infecting him or worried
for myself, but it was hard to focus when he began talking about
the results. I was trying to read the paper at the same time I was
listening to him, all of which guaranteed my failure.

"I'm lost" I said finally. He leaned over and used a pen to
point out the result he was speaking about. He did this with the
firmness of a tutor who thought his student capable of understanding but for some reason wasn't. In my vulnerability, that
little girl who lives inside of me came to the fore and thought
for a moment, *Hmm. . . . This man could get impatient with me,*
a further distraction. But after he clarified the meaning of some
of the medical terminology, we made it through the report, and
I relaxed.

He had taken photographs of the inside of my abdomen
during the surgery and had shown them to Erik. We looked
at them together now as he pointed out the areas where there
were visible neoplasms.

"There isn't a lot of visible disease at this time, but we can't
just ignore what is there," he said. "Right now, you have options.
We can continue to monitor with CT scans and blood tests,
and then, at some point in the future, you could again consider
having the CRS/HIPEC treatment." He paused and made eye
contact with me. "On the other hand, it also makes sense to go
ahead with the surgery now, when there is a smaller volume
of disease to deal with." He paused and his tone became more
personal. "If you were younger, I would recommend that you
have the surgery, but at your age, it is up to you to decide what
you want to do. I am comfortable with either choice."

I was silent while trying to take in the fact that I was at the
point where the CRS/HIPEC procedure made some sense.
I assumed that the risk for my age group was why Dr. Adam
had given me a choice of options, rather than recommending
I do the treatment, but I didn't ask him that question.

He went on, telling me he thought I was a good candidate for the surgery despite my age. He went through the procedure, describing it step by step, and then revealed a long list of possible complications, some of them life-altering, even life-threatening. As I listened, I remembered my reaction after watching the CRS/HIPEC video. That day, I had closed my mind to all of it, tossed that procedure into a heap with other life experiences I couldn't bring myself to imagine. I didn't want to think of it ever again. Here I was now, with light shining in that dark corner of my mind, only this time instead of a video, there was a real, live, warm, caring person guiding me through this proposed process. While I could barely bring myself to think about it, here was someone who could talk about it as a real possibility, who could think about it in regard to me. Not only that, but he had experience doing the procedure. He had watched people go through it and watched as they came out the other side.

The relationship between a doctor and a patient is an amorphous thing. Often it is only imagined in its absence when neither the doctor nor the patient are capable of finding a connection, but I was experiencing the opposite. I was developing a deep trust in this man. On this day, that trust made all the difference. I felt like Dr. Adam had brought a gift into the room, one that looked pretty ugly to me from the outset, but something about the way he held it and offered it to me, allowed me to open to its possibilities rather than turn away. It was an offering, and now there was a choice to be made.

"So do you want to choose option one or option two? You can think about it and decide. As I said, I am comfortable with either choice," he told me. There was no pressure. I tried to speak. I don't remember my exact words, but in extremis once again, I fell back into an earlier version of myself. This time I wasn't a young girl. I was speaking as a young woman who didn't yet stand in her own power and perhaps looked to the patriarchy when decisions were tough. I muttered something that was a feeble attempt to get my answer from Dr. Adam. He looked at me, and with a voice full of patience and compassion, said, "It is something only you can decide." Embarrassed to find that younger woman at the helm, I stepped back into my wise-woman older self and left my appointment with much to consider.

I've never been one to want heroics in the face of death. Over my life, I had developed a deep trust in the natural processes in life, especially in the process of birth when I brought my sons into the world. I wanted to trust that when my time came to die, I could peacefully let go. I suspected that many who were my age might be ready to surrender to life's end, but I learned that I was not one of them. I'm not sure exactly how old I imagined myself being before I could join them, but it became clear to me that 75 was much too young for me to do so.

I've heard many proclamations from friends in their later years, say 65 and up, about how they would refuse treatment if they had a life-threatening illness. I've always found those declarations a way to feel in control of an uncontrollable situation. Their words sounded hollow in the face of a force far more powerful than our imagined ideas about who we are and what we might do. I have preferred to leave it as a mystery, believing that none of us knows what we would do unless we are actually faced with that decision. Here I was now, looking for my own answer. I found myself caught in an impossible space, somewhere between yes and no. I didn't feel ready to die, but my fear of the treatment was enormous. The thought of how much suffering I would have to endure was daunting.

Over the next few days, I sincerely questioned my ability to endure such an extensive procedure at my age. Yet, if I didn't opt for the treatment now, I would only be older when I faced that possibility some time in my future. I worried that I would be less resilient with each passing year. On top of that, the level of my disease would be more advanced. With that reasoning, it seemed clear that my best chance to deal with the surgery would be to have it sooner rather than later.

Further tipping the scale towards "yes" was the thought that at this stage of my life anything could happen to me health-wise. My diagnosis had come out of nowhere, ambushing me when I least expected it, like the airplane penetrating the wall in my dream. Things like this were happening to friends and family my age as well—a heart attack here, a lung problem there, a life-altering stroke. So many things could happen. If whatever it was I might get didn't kill me first, it might leave me no longer a candidate for the surgery. Right now, I was in control. I was sitting in that pilot's seat, looking at the control panel, and I could choose. The thought of that choice being taken away from me sent me down a dark alleyway in my mind. My brother used to tease me about my more cautious approach to life. *He who hesitates loses*, he would say with a snicker. He had been right about that more than once in my life. Here I was, again fighting with hesitation.

I remembered Dr. Adam telling me that LAMN wasn't such a bad diagnosis to have. It still seemed pretty bad to me, but I did realize that it wasn't like having ovarian cancer, which was my original fear. "Everything is relative in this life," he had told me. I was sure that Dr. Adam knew what he was talking about, since in his specialty, patients in tragic circumstances must come his way often. Yet, after being so healthy for so many years, even with two surgeries in the last nine months, I was still shocked to have anything at all wrong with my body.

It started to creep into my reality that I should be grateful there was a treatment for my disease, a treatment that could add years to my life. When I imagined something happening that would disqualify me, I felt lost and alone, as if I were wandering through a dark passage without a speck of light, all hope lost. All of this left me tipping towards saying yes to the CRS/HIPEC procedure and doing it now rather than later.

Calling Forth My Own Inner Healer

I never make my decisions based on my rational mind alone. There is so much more of me that wants to be heard. I've come to trust the wisdom of that older, deeper part of myself. Around this time, I had another powerful dream.

I am having a confrontation with an adversary who means me great harm. We are in a physical fight. I aim a blow in my adversary's direction, but it doesn't reach its destination with full force.

I woke up abruptly, my body shaking and my heart pounding. It took me a moment to realize that I was safe. When I calmed down, I was pretty sure that my dream was commenting on my health situation. In that arena, I was indeed struggling with an adversary that could bring me harm. The fact that I was taking aim, but my blows weren't striking with full force seemed like a calling to bring more of myself to my healing process. I wrote in my journal that night that I wanted to call forth my own inner healer and dedicate myself to making art about my medical situation.

The first art that emerged focused on the appearance of a brightly colored circle. The orb was rising from a watery base.

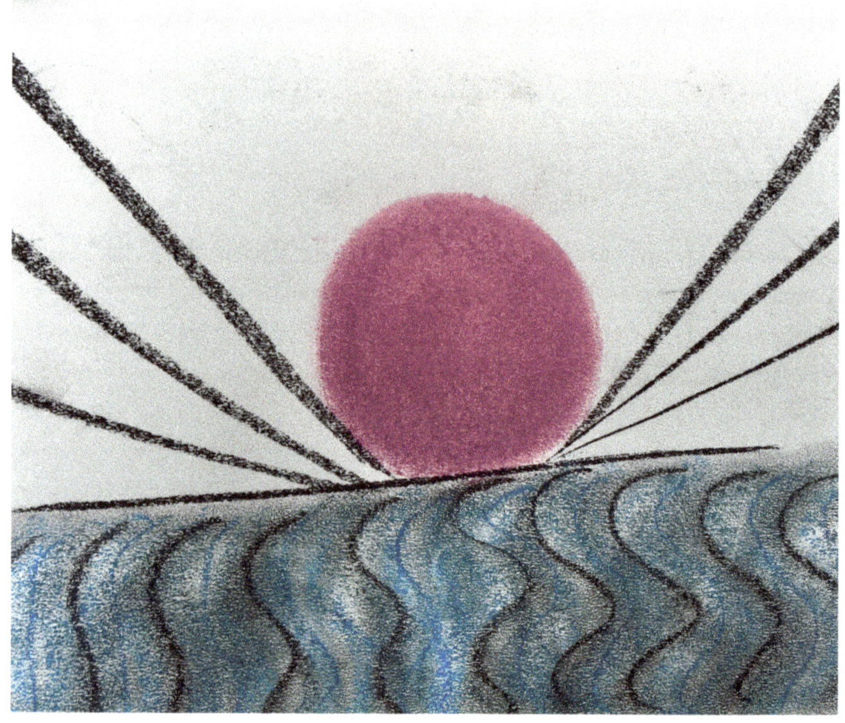

My Will to Live Rises

It was a simple drawing that I left out on my table so I could let its meaning reveal itself. Over days, I saw that fuchsia circle as my vibrant living self, rising from a watery landscape and being supported on the surface by those black lines. My attention focused on the dynamic between that fuchsia ball of life energy and the watery depths below. The black lines looked like they were ropes holding the orb on the surface, keeping it from sinking back down. It had risen from the depths and was being held there as if wanting me to be sure to see it.

The more I felt the possibility rising within me of saying yes to the treatment, the more I saw that fuchsia ball in my drawing as my will to live, rising up from the depths of my unconscious mind, the black lines insisting that I see it there fully exposed. I knew I had the will to live, but when not confronted with life possibly ending, that will can rest in the unconscious, supportive but not fully revealing itself. Here it was now, insisting I focus on it.

All this circled round in my mind when suddenly one day, as I was doing the dishes, my choice revealed itself to me. In my gut, I knew I would proceed with the surgical treatment. It was as if my body had made the decision. There was no point in arguing, though I realized my mind might try. I now knew what was going to happen. I would opt for the surgery because despite what I might have to endure, I was hungry for more life. It was as simple as that.

Imagine me making that decision at 75. Ridiculous you say? Well, that is what I said as soon as my decision was made. *No, this can't be!* an inner voice shouted in rebellion. *You are old! You have lived a good life, enough is enough! You are coming to your end. Accept that!* But my will to live was louder, boisterous even, and insistent, and once it rose up, it was not going to be easily stuffed back down.

My body was shouting, *yes, yes, yes!* My mind became increasingly desperate, perhaps because it could feel I was losing any grip I might have had on saying no. In a last-ditch effort to bring me to my senses, my mind called up the "good girl" who still lives inside me. Not wanting to be selfish and always being certain to put other's needs before her own, she chimed in. *Are you being greedy to want more life?* she asked in her little high voice, as if more years for me might mean fewer years for someone else. She was so insistent and sincere with her inquiry that I listened.

Did I really have the right to ask for more? Was I just being overly entitled? Should I be surrendering instead of jumping into action?

In my struggle, I confessed my dilemma to my insightful friend Tansy who is an Episcopal priest then in her eighties. In a spontaneous moment she quipped, "What? Do you have something against us old women? You think we don't have a right to live?" This sent us both into peals of conspiratorial laughter. That laughter with my friend ended any hesitation that may have remained.

The next day, I sent a message to Dr. Adam telling him I wanted to proceed with my surgery. The sooner it could happen, the better. I never questioned my decision again.

Chapter 6

Chipping Away at The White Coat

When I was healthy, I found it easy to have a good relationship with my doctors, but the vulnerability that illness brings upped the ante. Now that I had decided to proceed with surgery, I felt challenged in a whole new way. I was about to put my life in Dr. Adam's hands and that required a new level of trust. I wasn't sure how I would be able to find that much trust, but I was determined to try.

This led me to reflect on the larger issue of the doctor/patient relationship in our medical system in general. It is a complex relationship that begs an answer to this question: In the short time they have together, how do two strangers find a relationship that matches the needs and the intensity of the medical crises being faced?

The Art of Healing

Medicine is a science, but it is also an art. As patients, we experience the art of medicine or the lack of it in the relationship we have with our doctors. When confronted with a health challenge, most of us want to have a doctor with a *good bedside manner*, an old-fashioned phrasing that has come to refer to a person we can relate well with as we confront an illness. I certainly wanted that when I needed help, but in our society we create a power dynamic that puts doctors a cut above the rest of us. Some of us even look to our doctors as if they are gods. Some doctors think they are indeed God. This perspective seriously complicates attempts at finding a right relation with one another.

In my vulnerability, the more I longed for someone I could trust to the degree that I now needed to trust, it became clear to me that a relationship involves two people, not just one. So I had to try to figure out what it meant to be a good patient in order to hold up my end of the bargain. Did being a good patient mean I needed to do whatever the doctor said, becoming a passive victim of my disease? Or did I have an important role to play in bringing about my own healing? Do we enter the medical world like climbing Mt. Olympus, paying homage to a god, or do we seek a more equal footing as we come together to try to solve a medical problem? I began to wonder if there is an art to being a good patient, just like there is an art to being a good doctor. In the midst of all the complicated dynamics involved, how do we find our way to the healing relationship that I believe most of us, doctors and patients alike, are seeking? I was surprised that my questioning sent me down memory lane.

The Problem for Doctors

One thing I know for sure, doctors are human beings just like the rest of us. I know this because I was married to one for 25 years. It wasn't easy being married to a doctor, because so many in my small-town projected God-like qualities on this man that I had to live with 24/7. It is tricky for the ego to carry all those projections without starting to believe them yourself. As I saw this happening from early in our marriage, I took it upon myself to be sure John knew that he wasn't a god in our home. He still had to do the dishes and help take care of the kids. He still had to relate to me like a fellow human being. His insistence on his superior position and my penchant for knocking him off his pedestal caused enormous disturbance over our years together.

I wasn't always battling. I had enormous empathy when I saw the emotional toll his work took on him. The strain was palpable when there were crises, keeping newborn babies alive until they could be flown to a Neonatal Intensive Care Unit, sadness when he diagnosed a child with leukemia or a teenager with a brain tumor, and God forbid, if a young patient died.

The long hours, the grueling call schedule, and a life of continually responding to emergencies all limited our own life choices. I was less understanding of these logistical matters as it always seemed to me that family came last. It wasn't easy being a doctor or a doctor's wife. There was plenty of struggle, but there were also lots of rewards. As much as I struggled, I too benefited from the rewards.

Doctors live their lives closer to the life/death door than the rest of us. Because of this, it seems to me that training in some kind of spiritual or philosophical perspective might help them find their rightful place in the big picture of things, but I'm not sure they receive much useful training in that regard. In fact, I'm afraid the opposite is so.

I hope things have changed, but I was there when my ex-husband went through medical school, internship, and a pediatric residency. I witnessed how his training sought to help him develop objectivity, a supposed safe space where he could care for his patients; retain his ability for objective analysis; and protect himself from overwhelm when patients didn't do well or died. Those were all completely understandable goals, but finding the right balance was like learning to walk on a tightrope.

Balance may have been the goal, but the teaching came while obliterating the humanity of those going through the training. Medical school, internship, and residency were not for the faint of heart. Basic human needs like sleep, time for meals, time with family, were all but ignored. It never made sense to me. Who would want a doctor who hadn't slept for 24 hours taking care of their hospitalized child? Young doctors in training seeking any semblance of a balanced life were just out of luck. If there was anything left of your humanity when you completed your training, you could try to pick it up when you were spit back out into normal life once again.

As I witnessed it, medical training was a crash course aimed at convincing you that you were something beyond human, that you were indeed a cut above. Perhaps the root of the "God problem" for doctors was right there in their training.

I could not do a job where I held people's lives in my hands. I know that about myself. As smart as I might be, as well trained as I might feel, as much as I might want to be of help, or as much money as I might want to make, I could not carry that much responsibility. The fact that my decisions or my actions could mean life or death for someone is to me unthinkable. There is no way I would be able to handle the misjudgments or mistakes I would inevitably make because I am not perfect. I am human, and it is human to err. I doubt that I could ever be trained to forget that.

I'll bet many people feel as I do in this regard. Whether we think about it consciously, or whether our gifts and talents lead us to other professions or other work, somewhere in the recesses of the mind, we know there is power in those who can accept the responsibility that doctors accept. There is power in people who are not only willing but perhaps even enjoy taking those big risks.

Doctors carry malpractice insurance to help them manage the risk financially, but what happens inside when things go wrong? I remember being at a social gathering with a group of young doctors and their wives. We had all just moved to the area, and the doctors, all men, were busy establishing their practices. Everyone was alarmed because out of nowhere there had been a huge rise in the cost of medical malpractice insurance. It was the worst for the OB/GYN doctors and the surgeons, but everyone felt financially challenged by this price increase. One of the charismatic young male doctors declared he was planning to "go bare," meaning he was going to practice without insurance.

This idea caught on like wildfire as everyone contemplated doing the same. You could feel the energy in the room building to a frenzy, and soon many were proclaiming they'd do the same. Then, an older man, a visiting professor from UCSF, rose and got everyone's attention. The room fell silent as he spoke to all.

"I can empathize with how you are all feeling," he said. "But let me be the voice of experience. I know you don't think about this much, but one day it is inevitable that you are going to make a mistake, maybe even a terrible mistake, and when you do, you are going to be so very grateful that there is such a thing as medical malpractice insurance and that you have it. It won't make up for your error, but it will be something that might help those you have harmed. So think about that before you make your decision." You could hear a pin drop in the room as all those young men came to the realization that they were indeed human beings.

I admire tremendously anyone who decides to enter the medical profession, but admiration can be a tricky thing because it provides a fertile ground for projecting god-like powers onto others. Perhaps the root of the problem of seeing doctors as gods starts here for patients and our society in general. Doctors are ripe for accepting our projections, and we are ripe for making them. Projections install doctors as gods on Mount Olympus, completing the job of ensuring superiority that began in their training.

The Problem for Patients

When I was married to a doctor, I saw the human being behind the God-like image, but as a patient, I was finding it wasn't so easy to make that human-to-human connection. That is because as patients, we have an investment in wanting our doctors to be a cut above. What they know and their skill in delivering it can have huge consequences for our physical wellbeing. When illness leaves us standing at that life/death door ourselves, coming into right relation with our doctors isn't any easier for us than it is for them. I'm afraid we are both part of the problem. The good part of seeing it that way is we can both be part of the solution.

The medical world can feel like a monolith dedicated to its own practices and requiring total submission from patients. When we try to enter that world, we often leave important parts of ourselves at the door. At the core of this problem is the issue of power, and who we allow to have it. Most doctors are comfortable with their power, many needing to turn over some of it in order to connect meaningfully with their patients. But I'm afraid as patients, we all too easily relinquish the power we do have, often without even realizing it. At least that was true of me when I started out in my healing journey.

But I was learning an important lesson: To find and honor my own authentic presence in the medical world, I needed to bring my whole self to my healing process. My rational mind served me well in gathering and processing information about my medical situation, but I also needed to open to the wise voice inside of me that knows a great deal about what I need to heal. I wanted to bring all of me to my healing journey, but I wasn't sure that all of me would be honored by my doctors and helpers. In fact, I was afraid I would be ridiculed.

It is easy to feel like a helpless child when you are facing the massive power of serious disease. As children, we count on others to take care of us. If we enter the medical world in this childlike state, we hand our power over to our doctors, seeing them as all-knowing, superhuman beings. *I'll just put myself in their hands. I'm sure they know what is best for me.* This is not a good thing for our doctors, nor is it good for us.

Becoming childlike isn't our only reaction. Rather than becoming vulnerable children and turning our doctors into gods, sometimes we choose to denigrate our doctors' medical knowledge and expertise. *Doctors don't know what they are talking about,* you might say. When sensing the power physicians have in the medical world (especially after you have given them all of yours!), you can become reactive and rebellious, behaving like a hostile teenager in an attempt to cover feelings of powerlessness. A sad example of this are the stories of patients with Covid who are in the hospital unable to breathe, near death from the Covid virus, still insisting they don't have it and furious at the doctors for thinking they do.

Most troublesome of all are those times when we go into denial. Understandably overwhelmed by the whole situation, it can seem like a relief to fall into complete passivity. Refusing to become a patient, you ignore or discount your symptoms until you are in serious trouble. Frozen now, you are unable to take any action at all.

Finding the Right Relationship

None of these approaches give us what we really want, which is an adult-to-adult connection so we can build a relationship of authentic trust. I have had my own struggles with the doctor/patient power dynamic. At one time or another over my life, I have fallen into each one of those defensive patterns. But when faced with a life-threatening illness, I acknowledged my vulnerability and took the risk of coming forward with my own healing power, not to be in competition with, but to join the team of those trying to help me. There was healing in finding that I belonged there.

I don't think I would have recognized my rightful place on my medical team had I not found my way to embracing rather than reacting to all that serious illness brings. It is not easy to remain present with the dissolution of your good health, but avoiding difficult feelings leaves you more vulnerable to collapse or reactivity, both of which serve to cloud thinking and keep you distracted rather than focused on your healing. Only in staying with all the feelings that accompany that dissolution, will you find true power.

Chapter 7

Going All In

On the way to coming forward with my own healing power and joining the team of those who would be helping me, I realized this: Doctors are trained to find a place within themselves where surgery—the cutting open of the body—is an okay thing to do to someone, but patients are not. When I thought about surgery in the abstract, I found myself capable of compartmentalizing it the way doctors must, but suddenly my surgery wasn't an abstraction—it was something that was actually going to be happening to me!

While I understood all the steps of the procedure, I found that the less rational part of me wasn't as quick to put it in a box that made it all okay. *What? You are going to cut me open and then cut things out of me? Then follow that by bathing my abdomen with toxic chemicals? You must be kidding? Sounds inhumane!* Those weren't my exact words, but that is the gist of how I felt. What became clear to me was that if this craziness was going to happen to me, I needed a human-to-human connection with the person who was going to be doing it. Yes, I wanted Dr. Adam to be a well-trained expert in his field, but

I also needed him to bring his capacity for human connection. I didn't know how to ask for that, but I did realize I couldn't ask if I wasn't willing to bring all of me to the relationship as well.

At the time I didn't really understand why this arose so strongly in me, but like many things that arise from intuition, it often takes a while before you fully understand what is behind your strong feelings. I've learned to proceed, trusting that over time more will be revealed. Only as I write now do I more fully understand what I was trying to sort out at the time.

If the compartmentalization approach to surgery isn't assumed, you realize that surgery is an incredibly intimate proposition. Human hands entering your body and interacting with your organs is perhaps the most intimate thing that will ever happen to you, and it happens with a stranger, not a lover. A conversation between my soul and the larger powers that decide whether I live or die let me know that on an existential level, I was ready to go ahead with this surgery. But as my awareness of the intimacy of the situation bubbled up into my consciousness, I knew I didn't want to be alone in my humanness as we proceeded. I felt that human-to-human connection was as important to my healing as the surgeon's expertise with the procedure. What was about to happen to me required a unique kind of compassionate connection.

Disease is a part of our human condition. Feeling called to help people who are ailing is a part of the human condition as well. I knew that that kind of compassionate connection between us holds a possibility for deep healing. I had experienced that possibility in my own work as an expressive arts therapist. My training was important, but I always felt that the bond formed between my clients and me was the source of the deeper healing.

The healing power of the universe is immense. I'm afraid we most often take it for granted. With major surgery in my near future, I felt I needed to consciously befriend that energy. If I was going to put my life in the hands of another person, I needed the magic of this deeply human response to be part of the experience. Something in me felt that if I could bring my healing capacities and stay connected to my deepest humanity and could be met by my doctor doing the same, a synergy would be created that could call in a healing power larger than either of us individually possessed.

Doctor Adam had told me that if I decided to go ahead with the surgery, he and his team would be "all in" to help me through it. Now I was coming to the realization that I needed to be "all in" as well. I couldn't just say yes and sign the consent forms. I was beginning to understand what it meant to bring all of myself to this process. I would not be coming to my doctor as a child saying, "Heal me." I would not be coming as a rebellious teenager fighting my helpers every inch of the way. I didn't want to fall into passive denial. I would need to step into my full power so my doctor, his team, and I could do this together. I knew I had to communicate some of these thoughts to Dr. Adam. I struggled mightily with how I might explain what I needed and wanted as we moved forward.

The Conversation

Time had marched on, and it was now mid-October. My friend Lindsay, a retired psychotherapist with whom I've had a deep friendship for many years, drove me down to the city the night before my pre-op appointment. In our hotel room, we listened to the poet David Whyte giving a talk about friendship. He made the statement that our true friends are the people who have forgiven us again and again. I have friendships that have lasted for 30 or 40 years now. There have certainly been ripples in those relationships, but my friends were coming forward in a big way to help me in this challenging time.

That night as we lay in our hotel beds getting ready for sleep, I talked with Lindsay about the things I felt I needed to say to Dr. Adam the next day. Despite all my insight, it was going to take courage. The closer I came to having to speak up, my own version of handing over power to the doctor was pulling me in that weaker direction.

"Maybe I should be more submissive," I said to Lindsay. "Certainly whatever he has to say to me is far more important than what I have to say to him." I was still confused about why it was so important to me that I reveal so much of myself. Though Dr. Adam had been kind and available in previous appointments, allowing time for every one of my questions to be answered, I didn't really know the man. I was stepping out in a way that I wasn't sure all patients did, and I had no idea how he would respond. Lindsay and I were both moved to tears when I rehearsed my talk with her. That was encouraging, as it validated for me that I was speaking from my heart, which was essential for what I wanted to communicate.

I got very little sleep that night, and when we drove to the medical center that next morning, I begin to think there wasn't enough of me present to have the conversation I'd hoped to have. By the time I was in the exam room, I was certain of that fact. I felt foggy and unfocused. Dr. Adam opened the door, and he, his physician's assistant Stacy, and a visiting medical student swirled into the tiny windowless exam room where Lindsay and I had been waiting. By the crinkle around their eyes and their buoyant energy, I sensed warm smiles beneath their masks. There were introductions all around, and Stacy opened the portal on the computer so that my son Erik, along with his wife Kristian, and my other son Eli could join our meeting remotely.

"I hear you are ready to go ahead with the surgery," Doctor Adam said as he sat down on a rolling stool. I nodded and said, "Yes, I am." He seemed pleased that I had made my decision. "I feel rock solid in my choice," I told him. "Good, good, that's important," he replied.

In voicing my commitment out loud, I felt the atmosphere in the room change. It was as if I had physically stepped onto a path leading to this major event in my life. There was no going back now, just a cascade of next steps until I had the surgery and then made my way through to recovery.

"I'm glad we are going ahead," he told me. "My team and I will be here to help you every step of the way. I want you to know that we will be treating all of you, not just your tumors, not just your disease." He paused for a moment. I don't know if he saw the tears welling up in my eyes. Then he spoke again, "It will help in your recovery if you can bring yourself to being all in with what lies ahead."

The room filled with a gravitas that felt like it was bursting with compassion. This profound moment in my life was being deeply honored. His words were going straight to my heart. I couldn't believe that what he was saying and what I wanted to talk to him about were all of one conversation. The warmth I felt was overwhelming. I let my whole body receive what was being offered. As I continued to take all of this in, my tears were brimming over. I remember breathing deeply and putting my head down as if I were receiving a blessing. I felt so genuinely cared for in this time of great need. It was humbling. I was experiencing a moment of grace right there in that exam room. The energy I had wanted to bring to this appointment was synchronously already there.

With that kind of beginning to our meeting, I knew I had to speak up and say the things I'd planned to say. If I didn't, I would be very unhappy with myself, and so I dove in.

"I have a few things I'd like to say. Would this be a good time?" I said tentatively, wondering if I could really pull this off.

"Yes, of course," he responded.

There was no turning back now. I had to speak my truth. Trying to control my tears, I forced my words to come. "You are asking for the very thing I wanted to say to you. I will bring all of myself to this process. I will be 'all in.' I promise you that I will be a good patient and do what is asked of me." I paused and then added, "If I err in carrying out instructions, my error will be in being too cautious," I said, knowing this part of myself well. "I might need encouragement in that regard."

He listened carefully as I went on. "I know you are a doctor, but I also recognize the healer in you. I recognized that in the person I sense you are, your warmth and your compassion, and in the way you treat me and my family. It's hard to express how important that is to me." I was relaxing a bit as I spoke, finding it a little easier to continue.

"I honor your education, your training, and your experience as well, and I am counting on that part of you a great deal," I said with a little laugh at what an understatement that was. I paused and took a deep breath before I spoke the hardest part of what I had to say. "I want you to know that I have a healer in me as well, and I will be bringing that healer 'all in' as we go forward."

There, I've said it, I thought. I felt confident to continue: "I am not a religious person, but I am deeply spiritual. I actually believe that if we both bring our best healing resource to this, we will be supported by a healing power stronger than either one of us can muster on our own." Dr. Adam nodded, but he didn't speak. He remained completely present and continued to listen.

Emboldened now, I turned to my friend and retrieved a copy of my book *Finding the Wild Inside.* I had spent seven years writing the story of the development of my inner life, complete with color photos of my artwork. "I'm embarrassed," I said, "but I want to give you a copy of my book. It just came out last year." Dr. Adam seemed surprised and a bit taken aback. "I want you to have it not because I think you should read it, but if you just flip through the pages and look at some of the art, you will know more about me than what you see as this gray-headed old lady sitting here in your exam chair."

I'm sure I was red-faced when I finished, but I was proud of myself for coming forward and saying all that I'd hoped to say. I still had some concern. He had said he wanted to treat all of who I was, not just my disease, but perhaps he didn't know just how much of who I am I was planning to offer up.

He evidently had seen my tears, as it is hard to hide tears behind a mask when all you can see are eyes. "Now," he said, "It's my turn to be emotional." He paused, looked down at my book, and then back up. "Thank you so much for this and for what you said. Your words are powerful and important. Even though I walked in the room saying those things I said, it is good to be reminded of their true meaning." He turned to the physician's assistant and the medical student. "Remember this conversation. This is important."

He held my book in his hands and told me that he would read it. I really didn't want him to. It wasn't necessary or appropriate. I knew I felt moved to give him my book, but I may not have understood my true purpose. I think now that it was part of my being "all in." As we were starting out on this arduous journey, I needed him to know who I was. My book held the story of the most important parts of my life. Symbolically, as I gave my book to him, I was placing my life in his hands. That is, after all, what I was doing when I said yes to having surgery.

I remember his finger gliding over the book's subtitle, *Exploring Our Inner Landscape Through the Arts, Dreams and Intuition*. He told me a touching story about his own early connection with art. "When I was a boy, there wasn't money for travel, so all the art I was exposed to was in books. I discovered the Mona Lisa, and I read everything there was to know about the painting and the painter, everything I could get my hands on." As he continued to speak, I couldn't believe the synchronicity. Here we were talking about art, something so dear to my heart. I would have never guessed that art would be the bridge we would cross in order to experience each other's humanity.

He continued, "And then, later in my life at the end of my surgery residency, we had to give a talk to our department. It could be about anything we wanted to talk about. I did mine on the similarity between art and surgery." I told him I would have loved to have heard that talk.

I was so grateful for being met in my attempts to reach out. Our conversation went beyond my wildest expectations. We were in this together. I felt I had become part of the team. I felt welcomed, all of me.

On The Ground

In the remainder of my appointment, I heard more about the surgery. An incision would be made from my breastbone to my pelvis, so that there would be sufficient access to my diaphragm. He would be looking at everything and would scrape away any tissue that looked abnormal. "I will have my hands on all your organs," he said. That stood out to me at the time, but he went on, saying he didn't expect my bowel to be involved, although he couldn't be certain. We would have to wait and see. The exploratory surgery had confirmed that I had a low volume of disease, but there was an area where there were adhesions from my hysterectomy. He would have to look carefully there. This was of big concern to me. I really didn't want to come out of surgery with an ostomy bag because of the involvement of my bowel.

He added, "I will remove the greater and lesser *omentum,* the fused folds that connect or support the abdominal organs, as those are sites where the tumors can come back." When everything visible had been removed, he explained that I would be temporarily closed up. In order to deal with the tumor cells that were not visible, chemotherapy would be put directly into my abdomen. It would be circulated by a pump and heated to 41 or 42 degrees centigrade. They would then shake or massage my abdomen for 100 minutes, a bit longer than that scary video had described. This would help the chemo reach every tiny crevice where the tumor cells might be lingering. I would then be opened up again, and my abdominal cavity would be rinsed. Because I had developed a hernia after my hysterectomy, a plastic surgeon would be called in to repair the hernia and make the final closure of my incision. The surgery would probably take about eight hours.

"We surgeons cause the pain, so it is our responsibility to treat the pain, " Dr. Adam told me. He assured me I would be given an epidural in my spine for pain control, so I wouldn't need narcotics in my blood stream. The epidural would go in before the surgery and remain for 5 or 6 days. I would receive fentanyl through the epidural. There was no concern of addiction to the drug, which is an opioid, since the time of use was short, and it would be going into my nervous system not my blood stream. He explained that he wanted my pain controlled because I would need to be able to walk the day after my surgery. Walking would be essential for my healing. Furthermore, I would have a *nasogastric tube* inserted through my nose and down into my stomach to deliver nourishment for 3-5 days, and no food until I was able to pass gas. Then I would be on a liquid or soft diet. He guessed I would be in the hospital for 10-14 days, assuming I didn't have complications.

That was a lot to take in, but it didn't make me waiver. I sat quietly listening as he went on to speak about the risks and possible complications. Like a teacher in a classroom, he wrote them on a whiteboard in the corner of the room while carefully explaining each one. There was a 5 percent chance of dying from the anesthesia if my heart took a hit, a 5-15 per cent chance of bleeding due to lots of raw surfaces. There was a 25 percent chance of a major complication that would involve intervention, such as an abscess, sepsis, things like that. There was less than a 5 percent chance of having an *enterocutaneous fistula*, a leakage from the intestinal tract coming out through the skin. There was less of a chance of that if the bowel did not have to be cut.

Dr. Adam presented all of this calmly but firmly and then said, "I'm telling you all of this because these are things you need to know and not be frightened by."

I piped up with, "Well, I think I wouldn't be human if those things didn't frighten me."

"Of course," he said, "but you need to not let the fear overwhelm you."

These were grave facts. It was sobering to hear them, but I could feel in my body how I could be fearful but still manage my fear.

My trust in Dr. Adam had increased tenfold during this appointment. I did not feel alone heading into such turbulent waters. I knew that Dr. Adam, his team, and I would all be doing everything we could to get me safely through this storm. I knew that friends and family were there for me too, and the immensity of that support couldn't be underestimated.

After hearing all the things that could go wrong, I was surprised to find myself with one more thing I needed to say. "I want all of you to know that if something goes terribly wrong in what we are about to do, and I don't make it through, I've had a good life. It will be okay with me." I wanted my sons to hear me say that also, to know how I felt. I know that doctors receive training that helps them handle the loss of their patients, but I wanted Dr. Adam, the human being, to know how I felt, too.

Dr. Adam told me they would coordinate with the plastic surgeon's office and get back to me with a date for my surgery. "The sooner the better, as far as I'm concerned," I said. He let me know that if there was a holdup, it wouldn't be because of his schedule. He, too, sounded ready to go.

If Something Goes Wrong

The next day, I was telling my son Gabriel, who had not been able to attend, what had happened in my appointment. I was careful to remember to tell him that I was at peace with my decision and would be okay if something didn't go as planned. As a National Park Service Forest Ranger, Gabriel's job had a law enforcement aspect, and he had received training to handle life-threatening situations. He listened to what I was telling him, and then he asked if I would like a piece of advice. This struck me funny because since my sons have all been adults, I have made it a point to always ask if they would like a piece of motherly advice before I offer it. I told Gabe that I wanted to hear what he had to say.

"About that last part—if something goes wrong," he said. "In my training, we are taught to think ahead about all the reasons why we want to stay alive, so that if we get in a life-threatening situation, we don't have to start thinking about it then. There isn't time. It needs to be in the forefront of our minds. Our survival depends on it. I would think it is the same for you, going through your surgery."

I was so grateful for his advice. He was right. I had many reasons why I wanted to stay alive, and yet it felt true that it would be all right with me if I died. We tend to think in opposites, but I began to wonder if it was possible to hold these opposite realities inside me at the same time. At 75, both seemed absolutely true. Maybe I didn't need to choose between being okay if I died and fighting with everything in me for my life.

An old mentor once suggested to me that we have two different alignments in our human experience. The world over, these two parts of us are represented by the cross. The vertical alignment concerns our individual souls and their relation to the larger forces of the universe. Questions about life's purpose and life's meaning are asked and answered on this alignment. *Why am I here? What is my place in the Universe? What shall I make of my life? What is mine to do?* Our horizontal axis isn't about our individual souls amidst the cosmic forces, but rather about our relationship with one another and all that surrounds us here on earth. When we are at our best, this is the realm of love, connection, and belonging. At our worst, it becomes a place of separation, disconnection, and isolation.

The Celtic cross draws a circle around the point where our vertical axis and our horizontal axis cross one another. It is a challenge to live our lives in that circle, at that point of intersection. There, we can bring the unique beings that we are into relationship with the world around us. Intersecting in this way, we find the place of our true power. While we can't expect to achieve perfect balance at all times, when we do, we discover all of who we are, our wholeness.

Gabe's advice offered me the gift of coming to my surgery inside that circle at the point of intersection. Being willing to do everything that might be needed to survive was about my belonging here on earth, my horizontal orientation. Knowing that I had a place in me that was okay with my life ending was an existential proposition. It might mean that my purpose for being here on earth had been fulfilled. Thoughts like these rested in the vertical axis of my life. My healing would come in that circle where those two parts of me intersected. A synergy there would determine the outcome.

Chapter 8

The Long Way to Permission

When I received the date of November 22nd for my surgery, my imagination went wild. Making note of it on my calendar brought a chill. This was really going to happen. To the physician doing it, surgery is a procedure, something they have learned to do. I, on the other hand, was astonished that such a thing was even possible. In fact, it was pretty much completely unimaginable, which is why my imagination jumped into service, trying to help me prepare for the inevitable.

I'm sure most patients don't react as I did, but I became curious about this thing that I couldn't even imagine. *How does someone take a scalpel and cut into human flesh?* It wasn't that I didn't know or understand what was going to happen in the surgery, it was just that I had a hard time imagining it happening to *me*. To prepare myself, I felt I needed to look directly at the fact that my flesh was going to be cut, the neoplasms would be scraped off my inner body parts, cut out when necessary, and then a poison swirled around inside my abdomen.

One way I knew to look directly at something that was difficult to see was by making art. My intuition popped in when one morning I awoke with the thought that I needed to draw a representation of myself, then use a razor blade to cut open my abdomen in the drawing. *Now that will be directly looking,* I thought to myself. I didn't know what that would look like or feel like, but I knew I had to do it. Intuition is often referred to as coming "from the gut," and I was going to have "gut" surgery. Mind and body couldn't get any closer. This idea validated my thought that using art, exploring my dreams, and paying attention to my intuition would be vital to my healing, the key to activating my own inner healer.

Operating on Myself

Later that day, I sat quietly, staring at the bright white piece of paper on the table in front of me. It is always a little intimidating to start a drawing when I have no idea what is going to appear. Because I come to art to learn what it has to teach me, I try to put my thinking mind aside and let my body do the art. In that way, I tap into my intuition and am more of a witness to the process than the one doing it. Sitting down at my dining room table, I watched as my hand selected an orange pastel from its slot in the box. Orange is not a color I use often and certainly not when I'm going to draw a person. But my intuition had made the choice, and I've learned to go with that rather than shout, *What? An orange person?*

When I saw the orange pastel in my hand heading for the paper, I immediately understood why I had chosen it. Dr. Adam had given me the photographs he had taken of my insides when he did the exploratory surgery. While I thought of my inner cavity as existing in darkness, a light had been shone in there to take pictures, making them appear pink, orange, and brownish red. Some of them reminded me of the Red Rock Country in southern Utah. Picking the orange pastel let me know that those photographs had turned my image of myself inside out. I was evidently now made of orange.

I wanted to move fast so my intuition didn't get overpowered by the technical considerations of trying to make a likeness of myself. I quickly drew some semblance of a head, body, arms, and legs and gave myself a face, a pretty intense face, I noticed. This let me know that a serious matter was unfolding. It wasn't important that the woman pictured there look like me. What was important was she felt like me when I saw her on the paper, and she did. My intuition had made the figure. My body recognized a truth about myself in what I had drawn. I titled the picture *Operating on Myself* and proceeded to follow where my intuition was taking me.

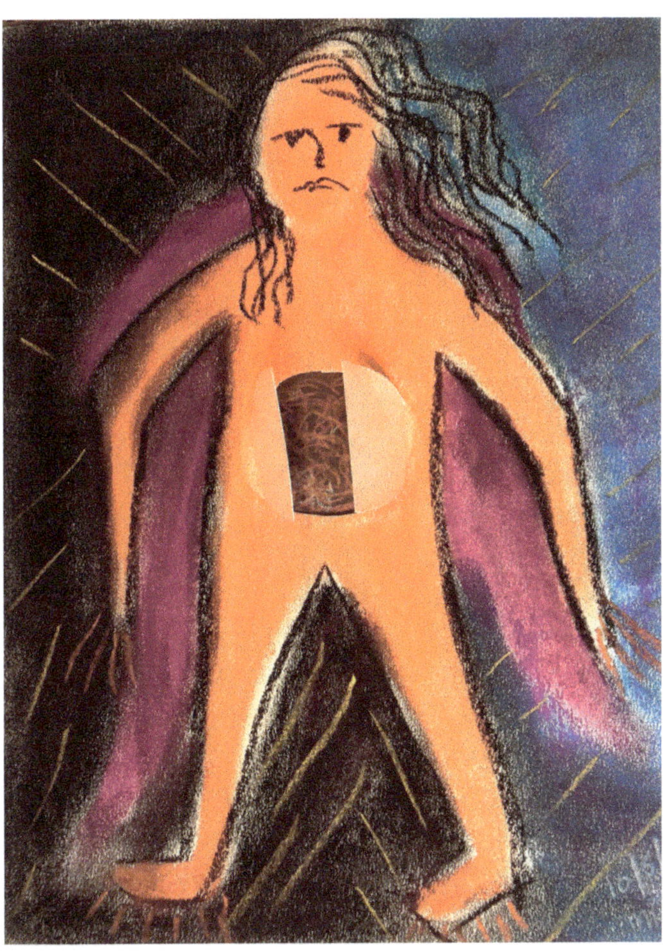

Operating on Myself

Once I had completed the figure, my hand went to the fuchsia-colored pastel in my box. I started to draw a cape which resembled wings and then ended up as just a fuchsia-colored energy behind me. I wasn't sure what it was, but I decided to just let it be. It felt supportive. Then I filled in the background starting with the black on the left and transitioning to the blue on the right. Lastly, I added the yellow lines. The movement from black to blue with yellow streaks let me know that my searching in the darkness was bringing some light.

Later, I noticed that the fuchsia color I had used behind me was the same color as the big round circle in my previous drawing, representing my will to live. It was comforting to see that it appeared here, as it was a major force in my decision to go ahead with treatment. Now I knew that my will to live would be a vital part of my making it through the operation. I was entertained by how this had all unfolded. I found a smile on my face as my picture had already taught me a lot.

Things grew more serious when I picked up a razor blade and prepared to cut into my abdomen in the drawing. It actually felt like I was going to be doing the surgery myself. What I was doing might have been called witchcraft back in history, but I didn't have a belief system framing my actions. I was simply following the voice of my intuition and allowing my imagination to grow really big. I was pretending, an important aspect of play, and letting myself go deeply into it. I was allowing myself to dissolve some of the boundaries between the world and my psyche, but I also had a strong witness inside that knew I was stretching those boundaries and therefore was not concerned.

My marks on the paper had taken me into what I call a *ritual art space*. I was aware of my little ego self who was sitting at my dining room table drawing, but I had an inner sense that something beyond little me was at play here. Perhaps because my conscious and my unconscious mind were in communion with one another, the world around me had grown enormously large. I loved the feeling of that larger world. Perhaps more importantly, I felt loved by it.

When I fall into a moment like this, I realize the power of art to take us deeply inside an experience. I had dropped into a magical space which is the closest I come to experiencing the world as our earliest ancestors perceived it, a world where our rational mind had not yet fully separated out from our animal nature and thus our place of belonging in Mother Nature. I say *the closest I come*, because we cannot go back there, but when our unconscious self and our conscious self are in communication through artmaking, we can experience a wilder mind.

It is a surprise to meet the part of us that existed before rationality became our dominant way of thinking. Some of us have a natural bent for living in this creative state, but everyone can learn to inhabit it. All it takes is letting your rational mind step down off its pedestal and allowing your body wisdom, your intuition, and your imagination to step up.

In this state of mind, I very consciously made a single vertical slit with the razor blade into the abdominal region of my drawing. Seeing it, I was confronted with the fact that my abdomen would have to be completely opened and accessible during surgery, so I had to allow for further access. I knew it wasn't what would happen in my actual surgery, but in my drawing, it occurred to me to make the opening a circle. I left just enough paper uncut on the sides, to serve as hinges, creating two little doors that opened and closed.

At first, I didn't really register the symbolic nature of what I had done, but later I realized that as I turned that vertical slit into a circle, I had symbolically placed the opening of my abdomen into a sacred context. My actions were reminiscent of that circle around the vertical and horizontal axis of the Celtic cross. This let me know that however my surgery would be held in the outer world, I would be holding it in a sacred circle inside of me.

Seeing the gaping hole when the little doors were both open, I instinctively selected a piece of black paper and glued it to the back side of my drawing. Now, when I opened the doors to my abdomen, there was something there. I drew the mucinous neoplasms that were causing my problem inside that dark circle, behind the open doors in my picture.

When I finished, I felt like I had completed an important task. With feelings of awe and wonder at what had been revealed in my art process, I sat quietly with my drawing letting all those insights settle inside me. I began playing with the little doors to my abdomen, opening and closing them in my drawing. As I did that, I sensed a different energy in my own abdomen. Paying attention to that new energy, I found that I was no longer thinking of surgery in an abstract way. I was thinking about it differently. My art experience had brought me just what I was looking for, a way to imagine, in a bodily way, what was going to happen to me.

A Deeper Permission Needed

When you agree to have surgery at UCSF, there are forms to be signed granting permission. They detail everything that might possibly happen in the surgery. Once I had decided to proceed with my treatment, it was no effort at all to let my pen glide across the paper with my signature, affirming my permission. That is what the doctors and the hospital need in order to proceed. I needed something more, a permission not given by my signature but from a deeper place inside of me.

I might not have known that deeper need had I not listened to that little voice on awakening that day, telling me to make art about my surgery. It would have been so easy to ignore it and just sign the requisite papers. Thankfully, on that morning I got the message. In using my own hands to cut into my abdomen in my drawing, I had come to terms with the cutting itself, and with that, I realized I had, in a very deep way, given Dr. Adam permission to make his cut into my actual flesh. I could now imagine it.

Leaving my drawing out where I could see it, I continued my relationship with the opening and closing of my abdomen. I played with the doors as I walked by, some days wanting them open and other days, knowing I needed them closed. It was a game. Sometimes it felt a little silly, but I kept it up anyway. I was exploring my feeling of vulnerability in regard to my surgery. Some days I could open to it, others not. My little game did make me think about my abdomen a lot, even when I wasn't looking at my drawing. I had a new relationship with it. It felt like a conversation that flowed throughout the day, as if to prepare that vulnerable part of me for what was coming.

An Epiphany

One day on my morning walk, this conversation surprised me by deepening into one of the more profound moments of my life. I had been walking along the cliffs above the ocean, listening to birds chirping their greeting to the day. As I walked along, I heard the waves roll onto the shore with a *whoosh*, and then make the rocky shore beneath crackle and rumble as the water rushed back out to the sea. It was like hearing the ocean breathing, one long inbreath followed by another long outbreath, repeating itself over and over again. Melting into that solid rhythm, I found my own breath deepening.

The sun was about to rise in the east, turning the water of the bay into the pinkish color of the sky. As the sun peaked over the hills, I felt its warmth on my face and watched how the early morning light danced with shadows when the breeze rustled the grasses on the headlands. But in the moment when I experienced my epiphany, I wasn't lost in all that beauty, I was circling back to my car by cutting through a residential area at the edge of my small town.

Walking along, I watched a man with a lunch pail leave his house, get into his waiting truck, and drive off to work. I heard the clanging metal of a garbage truck a few streets away on its early morning pickup route. Town was starting to stir, to wake up and join the day. It was all very ordinary, and then it wasn't ordinary at all.

In my imagination, I was suddenly aware that my abdomen was wide open, not like in my picture but graphically with my organs exposed. That moment in my pre-surgery appointment when Dr. Adam had said. "I will have my hands on all your organs," had stayed with me. That morning, as I walked down the street, lost in the story that was unfolding in my imagination, I was surprised to feel a human hand reach inside my body and make contact with my internal organs.

I instantly burst into tears. Fortunately there was no one there to witness this, as they may have been concerned. What went through my mind was, *Dr. Adam, when you make contact with my organs, please convey my gratitude for how impeccably they have served me for all these 75 years.* I felt like I was grasping the miracle of life as it moved inside my own body. My gratitude was instant and overflowing.

It took me a moment to recover. When I did, I couldn't get that feeling of being touched, where I had never been touched before, out of my mind. *What would that be like for me in my surgery, for my organs?* In that magical moment, it was the gentlest of connections, and yet it felt profound. How does one touch something that has never been touched before? It was as revolutionary as the first human stepping onto the unexplored territory of the moon, or perhaps how I felt holding my newborn infants for the first time. Such love in that meeting, such reverence for life.

The hand reaching into my abdomen was coming to heal, to nurture life inside me. There was such beauty in that gesture. Love saturated this entire experience, love for the miracle of life, love for the kindness of this helping hand, and a whole new love for myself, as if revelation of the perfection of life functioning inside of me had wiped out any question I might have about my self-worth. From inside the miracle of life where I had been for that fleeting moment, everything was love. I was humbled by the experience.

When I returned home, I knew I needed to turn to art, to make some attempt to express something about what all of this meant to me. I chose a sheet of black paper for this drawing as the revelation I had experienced felt as if it arose out of darkness, a moment when the Great Mystery revealed to me something about the essence of life.

My drawing started with the sacred circle of my previous drawing, filled with the colors of this newly revealed, unexplored territory of my abdomen. Next, I placed the hands reaching out to make contact. While these hands represented my surgeon's hands, they also represented my own hands, coming close and touching something essential about the nature of reality.

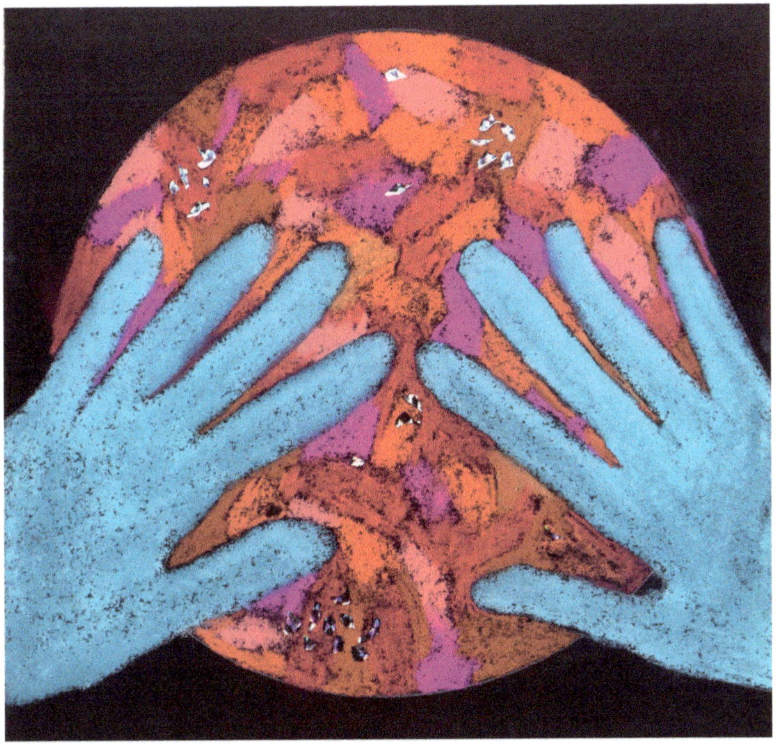

Touching *Gratitude*

I knew I wanted to picture the neoplasms that were the cause of all this exploration, but I wasn't sure how I wanted to portray them. I went out to my yurt where I keep my art materials to survey my supplies and brought back several items that might work. Back in my house, I tried one thing after another before settling on some bright shiny pieces of foil wrapping paper. I cut the paper into tiny pieces and scattered the pieces throughout the area of my abdomen. I was playing now, as I glued them down, wondering if making them so sparkly was some attempt to light them up so Dr. Adam would find every last one of them. Suddenly this deadly serious surgery took on the character of a treasure hunt, and that made me laugh. When I can laugh at deadly serious things, I know I am close to the place where my deepest healing resides.

As I sat with my picture, the little flecks of foil kept jumping out at me. They looked like little jewels. My attention was then drawn to the hands in my drawing being my own hands, as they seemed to be touching something very essential and profound. I realized that since my diagnosis, I had spent most of a year wandering through unexplored territory, seeing and experiencing things I had never seen before. While I wouldn't have chosen this particular exploration, I was discovering jewels of wisdom that may not have come to me any other way.

As I lived with my experience and the art that I had created, it was the love at the core of everything that was the overwhelming message. I had come to imagine my surgery with far more depth than I thought possible. Who would have thought preparing myself for surgery would lead to such a deep lesson about love? I was left with a feeling of deep peace.

A New Framing

That sense of peace made it impossible for me to view my condition with any war-like images, so commonly evoked medically when referring to the disease process. I did not see myself fighting a battle against my disease. I did not sense that my body was an enemy, betraying me by producing the invading neoplasms. Most importantly, I did not see my surgery as a "search and destroy" mission.

If my surgery wasn't that, then what was it? Thinking about that, a sweet memory came to me. Years ago, I was having trouble with mice in my garage getting into my Prius and wreaking havoc with the wiring. Not wanting to kill the mice, I had set up a Have-a-Heart trap so I could catch them live and deposit them elsewhere in the forest. One morning, on my way to walk with my friend Joan, I saw a mouse in the trap. We were going to walk down by the river that flows into the ocean at the base of my town, a perfect place to release my little captive before we walked.

Once there, I opened the trap door and tried rather aggressively to get that tiny creature to come out. It didn't move. I tipped the cage trying to dump the mouse out. I banged on the top, trying to scare it out. Nothing worked, the mouse wouldn't budge. I was getting frustrated. My friend, who has a kind heart and a special relationship with all animal life, offered to help. She quietly knelt down by the trap, and in the softest, sweetest voice, she convinced the mouse to cautiously step out of the trap and mosey off into the surrounding plant life.

I was so taken by her respect for the mouse and her gentleness. It was a lovely thing to witness and left me a bit ashamed of my aggressive attempts to free the mouse. It was the gentleness of her coaxing that brought that memory to the surface. It recalled the gentleness of that touch as I experienced it on my morning walk. I thought about the neoplasms in my abdomen. Could I imagine them being gently coaxed out of my tissue in the surgery? Could I lovingly release them?

I started to see my surgery as a loving correction of a bodily process that had somehow gone awry. I didn't need my doctor to see things as I did. His gift was using the scalpel. His presence communicated his desire to help me heal, and I completely trusted his expertise. I had promised that I would bring my own healing potential to my treatment plan. I hoped I could help my cause with my vision of the situation. Inside me everything about my surgery was framed in love and gratitude.

I was amazed how, by just listening inside, my own inner healer was helping me to prepare for what was going to happen to me. All I had to do was listen, be aware of what was going through my mind and body and dedicate myself to take action on what was being offered. I trusted what was arising because it was leading me to love and gratitude. This is a good place to say that I am not naïve enough to think that everything that arises from inside we humans is positive and for the good. Much harm can from following a dark voice aimed toward separation and hatred, but with the open heart as our guide, there is safety. I kept listening, and it appeared that the next step in my preparations had to do with coming to terms with the chemotherapy part of my treatment.

Welcoming Chemo

I've lived my life trying to take good care of myself. I wasn't a fiend about it, but I paid attention to what I ate and what I exposed my body to. I was relieved to learn that my treatment wouldn't involve systemic chemotherapy, but I wasn't thrilled to think about the hot chemo being swirled through my abdomen for a hundred minutes, either. I didn't want to think of it as a poison that might harm me. I wanted to find a way to welcome it, to allow it to do its work and receive its healing properties. I turned to art once again.

I drew a torso so I would have a close-up look at my abdomen. I made a circle in that area that I colored blue and marveled that the cord through which the chemo would enter my body trailed upward. My hand had just taken it there. I wasn't sure why. Fuchsia entered the picture, this time in my loins, which felt like a good place for it, giving my will to live a place at the base of it all.

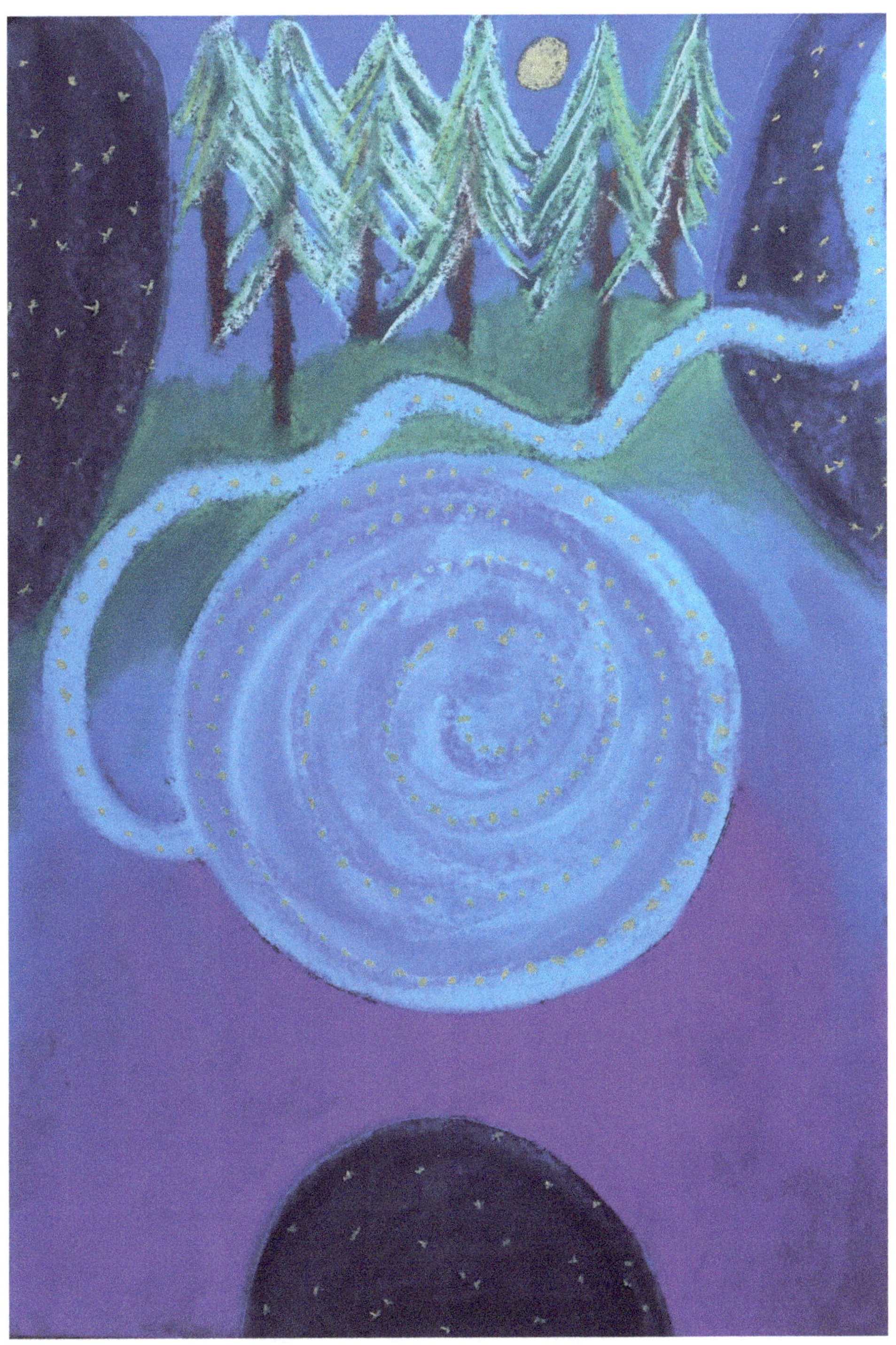

Swirling Chemotherapy

Next, I drew trees and a moon to represent my forest home in my chest area. I would be in the hospital, overlooking the San Francisco Bay, but I wanted to take the peace of my home in the forest with me when I went. I put the stars on the black paper around me, placing the chemo process under the mystery of the night sky, a place that has captivated me since I was a tiny child.

Following that, I spent a lot of time swirling colors around and around the blue circle in the center. I swirled and I swirled, and I swirled, until I was tired of making the motion and was pleased with what I saw. The tiny yellow dots were the final touch. Perhaps those little glimmers of light in the darkness were coming down through the tube to help me heal. Again, I was just letting my imagination play as I saw the drawing take shape. Then I knew in my gut that my drawing was finished.

Once again, my art had expanded my vision, placing this process in a cosmic perspective. If I were traditionally religious, I might have called my drawing a prayer. What it did for me was silence my fear of being invaded by a hostile substance. That cosmic perspective made me feel very small in the big picture of things, small, but a vital part of it all. I saw the tube coming into the circle in my abdomen as an umbilical cord connecting me to the heavens. The last verse of the song *Twinkle, Twinkle Little Star* begins with these lyrics: "As your bright and tiny spark/ Lights the traveler in the dark/ Though I know not what you are/ Twinkle, twinkle, little star." Perhaps those little stars in the background were coming out of the heavens and down that umbilical cord to guide the chemo into all the places that it needed to go to bring about my healing.

Resting in the Cosmic Egg

Weeks had gone by, and the time for my surgery was drawing closer. I was pleased with all I had done to prepare myself in the deepest way I knew how. I didn't know it then, but more was to come. How it happened surprised me.

Listening to the news one morning, I heard that a female condor at the San Diego Zoo had given birth to two babies without the help of a male mate through a process called *parthenogenesis.* Twice, the female condor's eggs had grown into chicks without being fertilized. They knew this because they had a DNA data base of all the birds in the zoo's flock. In doing some other research, they stumbled on the fact that these babies had the exact genetic material of their mother, thus proving what some referred to as their "virgin births." Parthenogenesis has been observed in nature before but in different species. When it happens, it is sometimes in extremis, when there are no males to fertilize the eggs.

I was completely taken by the story. It seemed a miracle to me and testimony to the power of the deep feminine energy to keep life going no matter what. I felt moved to make some art expressing my awe that this condor mother managed to produce those offspring all on her own. *How could that be?* To me there was more here than a biological fact. The story carried secrets of wily Mother Nature and the as yet, unsolved mysteries of life here on our Earth.

At the time, I didn't know that my fascination had anything to do with preparing for my surgery. I thought that process was finished. I Just knew I was completely taken over by this story. It brought me a deep sense of joy and celebration that life could carry on in such a way.

When I sat down to make art, I had no idea how I wanted to portray all I was feeling. I selected a black piece of paper once again. I wanted to start with this magical creature. I spent considerable time looking at pictures of these big birds, and uncharacteristically for me, I tried to make my bird look somewhat like a condor. I couldn't resist giving it a fuchsia glow in its chest area. There was that color of my will to live again, this time expressing warmth in the heart of this majestic bird.

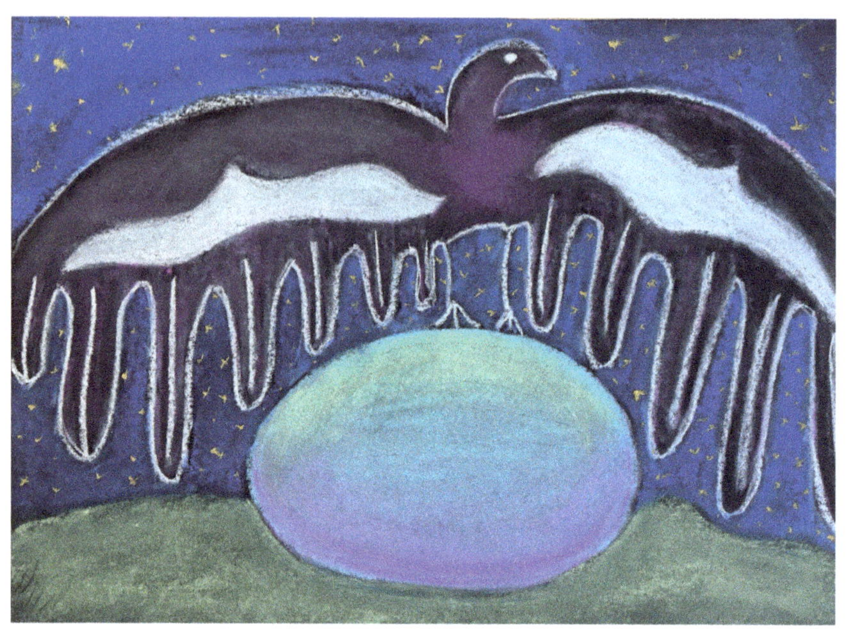

Awaiting Rebirth

When I placed the giant egg under the bird, I wanted to express its magic. I spent a long time blending the colors of the egg until it pulsated with the promise of new life. Soon I began thinking of it as the Cosmic Egg, a major symbol in creation myths occurring in all parts of the world and holding the mysteries of all life. Moving on, I colored the heavens a deep blue, gave it stars, and then embedded the egg in the velvety green of our earthly mother.

When I was finished, I felt my drawing said something about the power, the magic, and the majesty that I was feeling inside. It made me shake my head and let out a little sigh of amazement. I felt this story of the condor I'd captured in my art was a spark from the Great Mystery. What it revealed spoke loudly about how much we don't know, and how much we will probably never know about our life on Earth. My strong response to that thought was, *Thank Goodness! How would we ever experience our awe if we knew everything? What would happen to our curiosity, our sense of adventure?* Not knowing is such a part of being human and brings us so many gifts. How could we ever do without it?

I left my drawing out on the table, getting a little jolt of joy from it as I walked by throughout the day. I could feel the potential in the Cosmic Egg. With so much of my focus going to it, I became curious to explore more about the Egg's meaning in ancient cultures around the world. I found that the Cosmic Egg was represented in stories the world over as the container of life-force energy out of which universes are created. The Egg has everything within itself to hatch these wonders. Incubation is all that is needed for its potential to come into being. In the old stories, incubation is often provided by birds or sky gods coming down to sit on the Egg. The Egg itself is very much of the earth. Symbolically, its incubation by a creature from the sky world speaks to the coming together of Heaven and Earth, or Spirit and Body. The more I read, the more amazed I was that I had located this imagery inside myself.

Thinking of the condor incubating its egg in my drawing, I wanted to know more about what early cultures living with condors thought of them. I found that the condor was revered and held an important place in stories and ceremonies in many of those cultures. It was believed to carry prayers high into the heavens because of its ability to fly to enormous heights. At the same time, because it was also a carrion eater, it was connected to death and dying. It was seen to offer powers of renewal to humans, and thus was very much associated with the theme of death and rebirth.

One day as I walked by my art, I looked at that egg and thought to myself, *When I am under anesthesia during my surgery, I will be resting inside that egg, held in the power of the divine feminine energy, and watched over by this ferocious black and white bird with a very warm heart.* The thought surprised me, but it felt just right.

This was a part of the surgery that I hadn't yet explored. I would be under anesthesia for 8-10 hours and knew there was risk from that alone. I recalled Dr. Adam warning me about this part of the procedure in the long list of things that could possibly go wrong. I was concerned about it, especially at my age. Unbeknownst to me, my art had provided the perfect image to hold my concern. I might not have thought it up with my mind, but something deep inside of me let it emerge. All I had to do was follow my fascination with the condor story and make art about it, as that is what brought me this great gift of deep peace about being under anesthesia.

Around that time, my friend Lindsay, who'd had numerous surgeries, remarked, "Under anesthesia, they take you as close to death as possible and keep you there without letting you lose your life." That was quite a statement! Whether it was true or not, my imagination leapt on her words. I knew that the Cosmic Egg held the massive potential to bring new life, but as humans, we also live with the knowledge that all that is created will one day pass away. The old cultures didn't see this the way we do, in a linear fashion beginning with birth and ending with death. Rather, they held life and death in the never-ending circle, where death and dissolution have within them the possibility for new life to emerge.

If I were to believe my friend's words, I would be spending hours under anesthesia very close to the life/death/life door, that place in all the old stories of the world where everything begins and everything ends in the never-ending circle of life. I had stood by that door when I gave birth to my own children, but it wasn't until I was present when my sister gave birth to her daughter that I associated birth with the far end of life as well. That night I watched my niece's new life enter, and at the same time recognized that I would stand at that same door when dear ones—I had my aging parents in mind—would exit this world. It was a thought that illuminated my mind, but it was also a feeling in my body that expanded my perception, giving me a momentary glance of the miracle of life's great cyclical nature.

Thinking about myself hovering at that door for several hours, I likened my surgery to a death/rebirth experience, the hallmark of an initiatory process. I knew that my surgery would be a transformative experience for me, that I wouldn't pass through such a challenging event without being changed by it. Once again, I was finding a symbolic context for what was frightening me, enlarging the frame around that fear, and giving myself room to hold it differently, less fearfully and more powerfully.

It was another synchronous event to have heard the story of the mother condor, just as I was thinking about my surgery as a death/rebirth process. Coming that close to the possibility of my death, the story left me knowing that during surgery and my recovery, I would be working with everything I have to tip the life/death/life door towards new life. I was holding my time under anesthesia as a time of resting in the power of the deep feminine energy, being held there until I awakened, reborn to new life. I would be giving birth to someone who had my exact DNA, but I would find myself transformed in many ways by what I had gone through.

I was deeply curious about who I might become.

Chapter 9

The Blood and Guts Reality

Now that I was including myself as a member of my medical team, I wanted Dr. Adam to know how I was preparing for my surgery. I was concerned that it was out of line to use the UCSF My Chart messaging system for this purpose, but I didn't know how else to do it. Each time I brought more than what I guessed the typical patient brought to their healing process, I feared that it wouldn't be tolerated—not by Dr. Adam, but by the online system.

One day, I threw caution to the wind. I sent three of my drawings along with brief explanations of my process by email through that system. I feared I might receive a reprimand or at least be told I was being excessive. I did receive an automated educational email about how to appropriately use the messaging app, but very soon after, I received an email from Michelle, Dr. Adam's nurse, welcoming my messages and letting me know that they found my preparation "beautiful." Her email was signed "from the ENTIRE team," which I took to mean Dr. Adam had seen my messages, as well.

I didn't want to come off as some airy-fairy old woman lost in her internal psychic space, not realizing what was ahead for her. I wasn't that person, so I was careful to include this note at the end of my message: "Dr. Adam, I know I still have to experience all that is ahead in the blood and guts of physical reality. I know it will be challenging, but I believe that holding my experience with this much context and meaning bodes well for my recovery."

Coming to Grips

It was the "blood and guts" part that began to dominate my thinking in the weeks before my surgery. I didn't know how much suffering there would be. Dr. Adam had been clear about the importance of treating my pain so I could remain active after my surgery. I was more afraid of the treatment for pain than I was of the pain itself. I had given birth to all three of my children naturally, without drugs. I felt I knew something about handling pain, but pain from surgery would be different than the pain of childbirth. I didn't know what to expect or how I would react. I wanted to be reasonable and not make myself miserable by trying to tolerate pain that I didn't have to experience. I had no interest in being a hero in that way, but I didn't want to be overly treated for pain either. I guessed I'd just have to wait and see.

I wondered what the days in the hospital would be like. I was expecting to be there for two weeks, which seemed like a very long time. My family and friends gathered round. The Covid rules at the hospital had relaxed since my hysterectomy, making it possible to have someone with me every day while I was there. I gathered art supplies to take with me in case I felt up for drawing. I knew that if all went well, I would just have to be able to eat and move my bowels before I could go home. Entertainingly, my psyche leapt into action to assist me

with this possible future issue. I laughed when I awakened one
morning with this dream:

Someone hands me an infant. I am holding the baby by supporting her neck and her bottom. Her diaper feels very squishy. I lift
her up, to peek at her bottom. Sure enough, mustard-colored
breast milk poop is squishing out at her legs and over the top of
her diaper. A prolific poop! It is all over my hand and squishing
up the back of the baby's shirt. I can even smell its sweet odor.

Amazingly, my psyche had brought me an experience of "first
poop," and I had to honor it. Laughing as a drew, I pictured my
intestines filled with precious "first poop," the title I gave to my
drawing. It was as if my psyche was playing with me. Could
that really help me when the time came? I wasn't at all sure,
but why not go along with the joke?

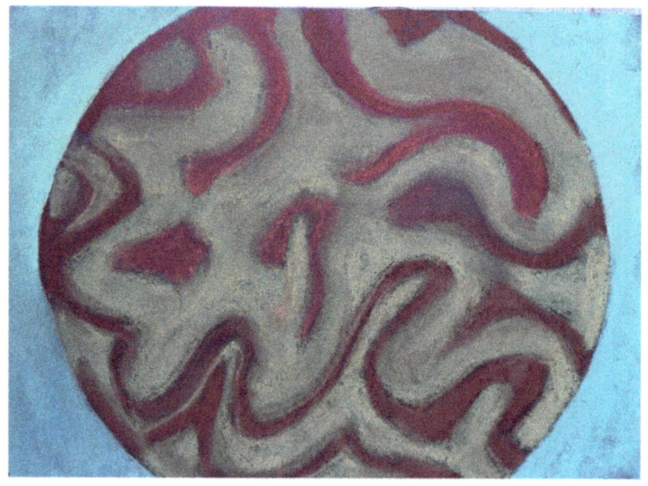

First Poop!

I was grateful for the humor of my first poop dream, but my psyche was also offering up darker matters. As the day of surgery neared, I had increasing thoughts about the place of suffering in human existence. The time was nearing for the physical wounding and the suffering that would be part of my attempt to heal. Surprisingly, since I'm not traditionally religious, images of Jesus on the cross came to mind. I mentioned this to my friend Tansy, the Episcopal priest whose wise commentary had been so helpful to me in choosing to go forward with the surgery. She lent me a beautiful book by Joan Chittister, *The Way of the Cross: The Path to New Life* depicting the path Jesus walked carrying the cross to Mount Calvary. The paintings were done by Janet McKenzie and were not the usual pictures emphasizing only the suffering of the Crucifixion. Instead, they pictured the women in Jesus's life and thus brought forward the compassionate response to suffering. The message that our suffering is also what brings compassion into our world helped me hold this whole dilemma.

I was also supported by the natural world as I moved through those weeks before my surgery. We had an unusually massive migration of brown pelicans visit our area. I love the pelicans and wait for them to come through every fall, but I had never seen anything like this. Their numbers increased over several weeks until there were thousands of them. At dawn and dusk, they covered every rock outcropping on the Mendocino headlands. On my dawn walk I could see solid lines with hundreds of pelicans flying to their feeding grounds where the river meets the sea. At sunset, they flew back in formation to the rocks for a night's rest. At their peak, I found myself visiting them morning, noon, and night. Everyone was coming out to see them. It was such a celebration, and it continued on for weeks.

Somewhere in the middle of this visitation, I came home from my morning walk, wondering what the old cultures thought of the pelican. Looking online. I was amazed to see that there were ancient stories of a mother pelican piercing her own breast to feed her blood to her babies if there was a shortage of food. The Christian Church picked up on these stories; the pelican feeding her babies her blood is frequently found in Christian art. Thus, the pelican has symbolized sacrifice and generosity.

It seemed I was surrounded with the theme of sacrifice and suffering. I drew a picture of myself with the pelicans to try out new iridescent pens I'd gotten for my time in the hospital. Looking at the picture now, I see that my shirt is reminiscent of the control panel drawing from my pilot dream. I like to think that I had fully embraced the pilot's perspective at this point in my medical journey.

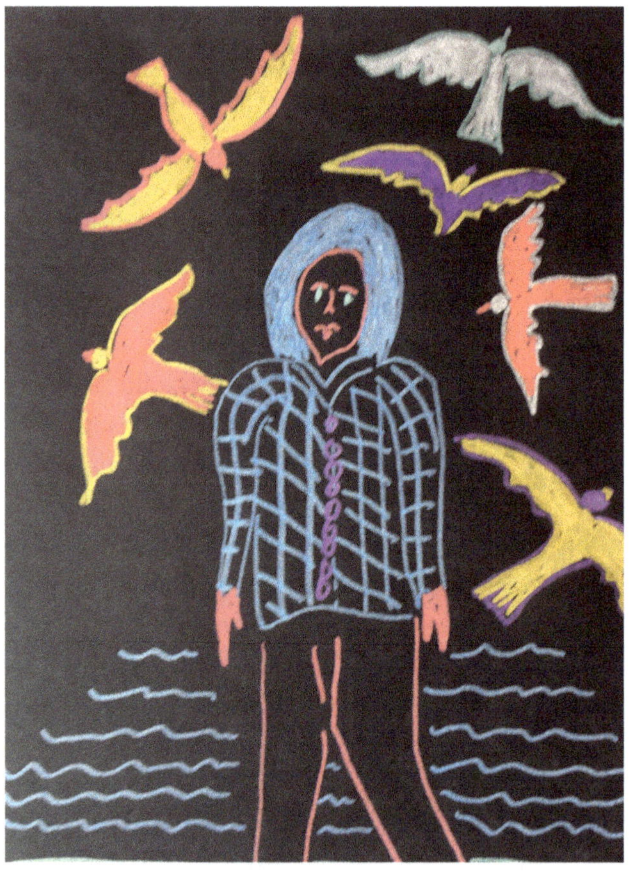

Pelican Blessings

The pelicans had arrived around the time of my exploratory laparoscopic surgery, eventually swelling into that giant flock. Then they began to fly off, so there were fewer and fewer each day. In the days before my surgery, every last one of them had moved on. It had come full circle. I was filled with the energy of the pelicans. It felt like a blessing.

There is nothing like a deadline to make you hyper-aware of time. That is how it was in the final days before my surgery. After all my preparing, internally I was surprised that I hadn't taken the earthbound step of checking to be sure Dr. Adam and UCSF had my Advance Directive for health care. This is a written statement of a person's wishes regarding their medical treatment, made to ensure those wishes are carried out should the person be unable to communicate them to a doctor. There was a last-minute flurry to get that on file.

Parting Gifts

I felt uncharacteristically optimistic about my surgery. I know when I was younger, I would have had much more fear. I wasn't thinking I was going to die, though I knew it was possible, but I was concerned about coming out of surgery with some sort of disability. In my imagination, a stroke would be a worst-case scenario or having something go wrong with my heart, but I was particularly focused on not wanting to have an ostomy bag. Dr. Adam didn't think that would happen but didn't deny that it was a possibility.

The day before I left home to go down to UCSF for the surgery, I woke up to an email from a friend who is a nurse. She had heard from a mutual friend about my surgery and my concern that if my colon had to be cut, I would need to have a colostomy. A colostomy is a surgical procedure that makes an opening in the abdominal wall. The end of the colon is brought through the opening and waste is delivered to an external bag, an ostomy bag. Her email let me know that one of her specialties was as an ostomy care nurse. She was trained to help patients learn to deal with the ostomy bag. She said she would be happy to help me if that should come about. She guaranteed me we could do it long distance and assured me that while it might be tricky at first, problems could be figured out, and we could find a comfortable solution. I was so grateful for her offer. This woman had moved away from my town, and I hadn't seen her in some time. Her message made me feel that I was in some way being watched over. Help was coming from unexpected places in unexpected ways.

I had so much support. Once again, Erik, Gabriel, and Eli came forward in a big way. They organized a Zoom meeting to discuss how they could help with my recovery. They put their schedules together and made a plan to rotate through my 2-week hospital stay, Gabe coming first, then Eli. Lastly, Erik would drive from Utah for the end of my hospital stay to bring me home. My friend Joanna arranged to be there when they couldn't. Other friends offered to come if my hospital stay was extended. Not only did my sons each plan to come while I was in the hospital, but they arranged their calendars so they could come to help me for a solid month after my surgery. The plan fell together easily as each one volunteered their best time to come. Because of work demands, at another time of the year it would have been impossible, but late fall made it all happen. I couldn't have been more lucky or more grateful.

My friend Joanna was my point person for communication. We made a list of friends who wanted to hear how I was doing during my hospital stay, and she offered to keep them posted. She also organized a list of people offering to come to the hospital to be with me and another list of those offering to help once I was home. As I packed my bag to leave the next morning, it was as if every single one of my concerns had been dealt with in one way or the other.

I had made this self-portrait. My torso looks like it has a curtain covering it, as if the curtain would just need to be parted for the surgery to take place. I was open, energized, and ready to go.

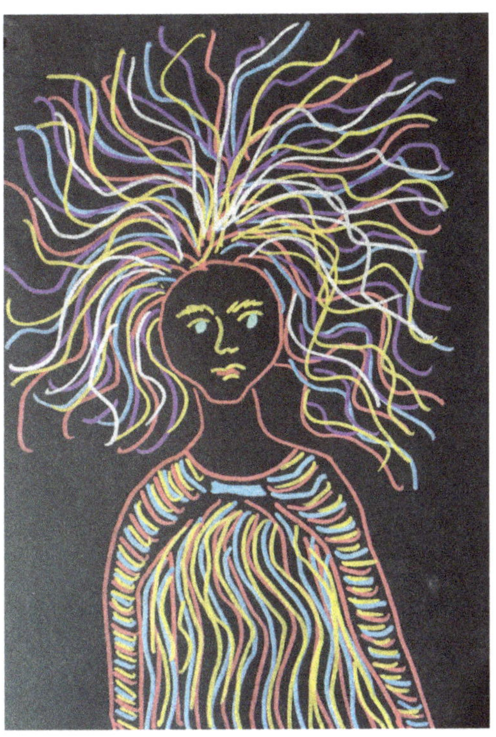

Wired

UCSF is about three and a half hours from my home. The plan was for Joanna to drive me to San Francisco and stay with me through the few days of surgery preparation. As I was doing my last-minute packing before leaving home that morning, I got a beautiful email from my son Gabriel. He was flying in to be there when I came out of surgery. I wept when I read what he had written. He commented on the "insight, perspective, determination, and strength" I bring to my life and how I had brought that to my healing process. And then he wrote, "I think your body is in the best, most capable hands in the world—your own, and that is comforting." He told me how much he loved me and that he couldn't wait to see me when I awakened from my surgery. I felt so seen by my son, not just as his mother but as a human being. His email built a bridge for me

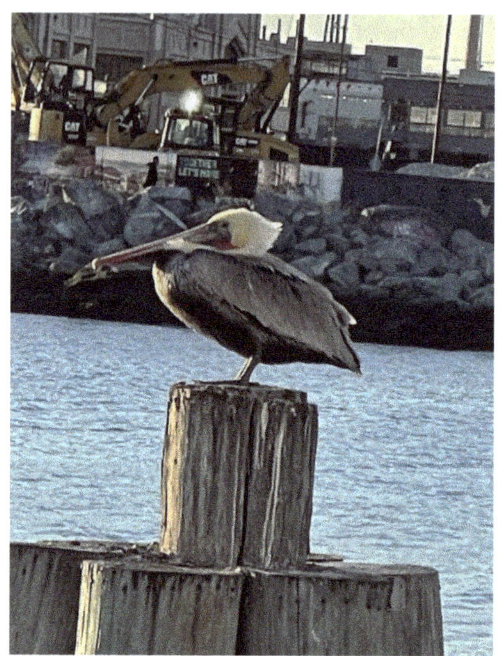

San Francisco Bay Pelican Messenger
(Photo Credit: Joanna Wigginton)

to walk across as I left home to go through all that lay ahead. I would see him on the other side of it all.

My friend picked me up. She had been present as a lay midwife when I gave birth to Eli at home, and now she was helping me midwife my healing process. Because I live so far away, we had to go down to San Francisco a few days early for Covid testing at a UCSF facility and then a full day of prepping for surgery. On my last morning of freedom, we spotted a pelican sitting on a post as we took a walk by the San Francisco Bay. Symbolically, the pelican was a signpost, a guardian, bridging my months' long experience of them at home to my time now at UCSF.

A Difficult Day

Considering what was about to happen to me, it might be surprising to hear that the prep day, a whole day before the surgery was actually the worst day of my experience. I had to drink stuff to empty my bowels. It was like prepping for a colonoscopy that I'd had recently, and my body memory was still way too strong to have to do that again so soon. I couldn't eat anything. I could only drink clear liquids which was not very appealing. Later in the day, I had to take drugs that left me nauseous. I think they were pre-surgery antibiotics.

As my nausea increased over the late afternoon, Joanna reached out to UCSF for help. There was a series of errors that would have been comedic if I hadn't felt so miserable. We were told to get an anti-nausea drug, but at the pharmacy we learned I needed a prescription. In trying to get that, I was told to go to the emergency room if I vomited too much but that if I went there, my surgery would be canceled.

It was getting late. Pharmacies were closing. The nearest 24-hour pharmacy was miles away. It was dark, and we were two country women not used to city driving. We felt helpless and hopeless. In our final attempt to get help, we never got a call back. I later learned that the doctor on call had called my home number rather than my cell. It was getting very late. I laid in bed desperately trying not to vomit. When I didn't succeed, I wept. After all I had gone through, I was fearful that my surgery would be cancelled because I had thrown up the medication. Sleep was scarce that night as I needed to be at the hospital before dawn.

The Big Day Finally Arrives

I had indeed entered the world of suffering. I was so grateful to have my friend with me. I couldn't have felt more supported as we made it through the hospital procedures and found our way to the surgical waiting room. I had heard from all my sons and had received texts from some of my friends. With almost no sleep, I was kind of dazed. At this point there was nothing but surrender happening inside of me. Time was speeding ahead. They called my name. I said goodbye to my friend and went through the double doors to the surgery area. My first words to Dr. Adam when I saw him were, "I threw up the medication!" His reply, "It's okay," melted the now seemingly unnecessary stress of the day before. So easily taken care of. We were going ahead.

I felt terrible, but I remained calm. I submitted to all the necessary preparation as many people came to do their part to ready me for surgery. They were a well-oiled team. I was pretty out of it from my lack of sleep, but I was present enough to convey my gratitude to each and every one of them, something that was foremost in my mind that morning.

I had read about patients requesting certain music in the operating room or asking their anesthesiologist or nurses to recite certain affirmations during their surgery, but I didn't want that kind of control. Now was the time for these professionals to concentrate on what they needed to concentrate on, to do what they were trained to do. I even felt that way with Dr. Adam. I had already made the connection with him that was important to me. On this morning, I wanted to give him all the space in the world to think about what he needed to think about in order to carry out our plan. So I submitted to what each person I met asked of me, marveling at the way they went about their work, and letting each person I made contact with know how grateful I was for them being there to help me.

Only now do I realize that I, too, was doing what I had trained to do. All my inner preparation had been about welcoming my treatment, trusting that by being open and receptive, I'd have the best chance to heal. The natural outcome of all my welcoming was my deepest gratitude to all those contributing to my cause. It was pouring out of me like a waterfall.

If there was fear in me, as I was wheeled to the operating room that morning, I wasn't aware of it. As the gurney slid down the hallways, around curves and through the automatic doors to the surgery area, I felt like I was floating down a fast-moving river, speeding to a destination I had been heading to for months now. When they wheeled me into the brightly lit operating room, there was nothing left of me but gratitude which I immediately expressed to everyone present in the room. The depth of my gratitude that day was palpable, not unlike the gratitude I had tapped into on my walk that magical morning some weeks before. I don't know if I was reading the room correctly, but the people I thanked seemed surprised, a little taken aback by so much gratitude.

This time was different than my past surgeries because an epidural had to be placed in my spine when I was still awake. They asked me to get off the gurney and kneel on a comfortable contraption, so my back was accessible. I wasn't terribly uncomfortable but was hoping this would go well and be over soon. I don't know if it was true, but I think maybe the first attempt didn't go well. I heard some words mumbled behind me. I saw a nurse quickly walk toward me from her preparations on the other side of the room. There was a shift of energy at my back as if someone else was taking over. I felt no pain. The nurse bent down and put her face right in front of mine. She locked onto my eyes as I did to hers and quietly told me to breathe, which I did, and it was suddenly all over. I was so grateful to that woman who seemed to be going the extra mile to help me with the sheer force of her ability to connect. It is a moment I won't forget.

They helped me back onto the operating table, making sure to let me know exactly what they were doing, placed the mask over my face, and I was gone. Where do we go when under anesthesia? I would love to know what we are experiencing. The body must know something, but I don't think I will ever know except in the bits and pieces that may filter through my dreams. I'm sure I was experiencing something, but it is lost in the mystery.

My son arrived in time for Dr. Adam to talk with him after his part of my surgery was completed. Another surgeon came in to repair my hernia. My surgery was 10 hours long. Gabriel evidently sat with me that night in the ICU, but I didn't know it. I don't remember waking up until the next morning.

When I opened my eyes, I startled Gabriel who had been staring at my closed eyes for so long. I saw the surprise ripple across his face as a big smile appeared. "Hello Mom," he said. Joanna was standing behind him leaning over his right shoulder. She said, "No ostomy bag!" I laughed inside. I felt celebratory. My new life had begun.

Chapter 10

Light-Hearted Marilyn

From the moment I opened my eyes in the ICU, everything struck me funny. I could see that Gabriel and Joanna were trying to assess how I was doing, and I wanted to let them know I was fine and found all of this hysterically funny.

I was not really in a funny situation. It took me a moment to realize that I couldn't talk as I was still on a respirator, and, as I'd been warned, had lots of tubes attached to me. In addition to the respirator, I had a feeding tube that went into my nose down to my stomach, and of course, a catheter to take care of my urine. All my bodily functions were being monitored.

I tried to write a message moving my hand in the air. They offered paper and pen, and I wrote "Happy, Funny." They laughed. I didn't think of it at the time, as I felt normal, but maybe it was the drugs I'd been given that were making me so happy even in these dire circumstances.

I saved those pages I wrote, trying to communicate with my loved ones that first day. Much of it is nonsensical or all jammed together and indecipherable. In my effort to orient, I did ask what day it was. I didn't know how long I had been out. I communicated that I was so happy to see them and thanked them for being there with me. I wrote that I was glad my mind was working as well as it was and that I felt like myself. I also communicated my needs: I was too hot. My throat was dry. Could I have some water?

My memories of my time in the ICU are fragmented. I have snapshots in my mind and remember what was happening in that moment, but there is no continuity of thought. For instance, I remember a resident doctor swirling into the room and standing over me.

"Do you have *a-fib*?" he asked urgently. I stared at him but didn't answer, thinking maybe he was talking to someone else. He asked again, "Have you had *atrial fibrillation* (an irregular heart rhythm that can lead to blood clots in the heart) before surgery?" Realizing he was talking to me, I shook my head no. "Well, you have it now," I remember him saying as he rushed out of the room. I wrote, *Who was that*? but I drifted off before I received an answer. My heart must have straightened itself out because *a-fib* was never mentioned again.

Later a nurse came in and said that she was going to weigh me. The scale was in the bed, so I didn't have to do anything. She asked if I wanted to know my weight, as if she didn't want to say it out loud with others in the room. I entered the hospital weighing 191 pounds, so when she told me I weighed 245 pounds, I was more than surprised. I wrote *Uh-oh*, and then it was all so funny to me, we women caring about how much we weigh. I wrote further: All women in America think about their weight until they die. My epitaph should be, "She thought about weight, and then she died!" This was very funny to me, but Gabe and Joanna looked concerned. I wrote, *Epitaph—JOKE!* They relaxed.

It turned out my weight gain was a reflection of all the fluids I'd been given during that long surgery. Early on, a nurse asked if I felt bloated. I said no, but later I looked at my hands. They were so round and puffy that the tops of both were perfectly smooth. The doctors assured me that my body would rid itself of all that extra fluid over time.

It was frustrating trying to communicate by writing, especially since I could see they were having trouble deciphering what I was saying. At one point, I wrote, *I wish I could talk.* This too struck me funny. Me, who tends to be quiet, wanting to talk? I wrote, *Funny when an introvert wants to talk!* I had so much laughter inside me, and I just wanted to express it. As I laid there hooked up to so many machines, so many things seemed completely absurd to me. Later that first morning, the nurse came in and told me they would like to remove the respirator. "Will it hurt?" I wrote. They didn't think so, and it didn't. I was so grateful to be able to talk again.

The main thing I remember about those early days in the ICU is that I had more than one reality happening at the same time. When my eyes were open, I knew where I was and who I was with, but when I closed my eyes, an entirely different reality was going on. Now and then, in opening my eyes, I would begin speaking from that other reality. When I saw the confused looks on my loved ones' faces, I'd realize I was back in our consensual reality. It was confusing.

When my eyes were closed, it wasn't like dreaming as there was no story or a plot line. It was just a slice of life going on in some other place, people walking down the street, people sitting around a table enjoying each other's company, me among them, though they were mostly people I didn't know and had never met. Once when my eyes were closed, I heard Gabe's sons, Chase and Cole, playing nearby. I was surprised to open my eyes and find them not there.

The physical therapist came on the second day of my ICU stay as had been promised. She taught me to roll over on my side and use the hospital bed rail to help myself get upright. I dropped my legs over the side, and there I was sitting up on the side of the bed. They helped me up, and I took a few shaky steps while she and the nurse cheered me on. They were surrounding me as I accomplished this mighty task and then helped me back into my bed. My walking had begun.

The miracle was that I was not in any pain, none at all. Dr. Adam came each day to check up on me. He was happy that I had no pain and told me that it was like that for about half of his patients. For others, not so much. I felt so fortunate to have fallen into this lucky half. Dr. Adam seemed pleased with how the surgery had gone. He had assured Gabe that I had made the right decision by going ahead with it now, rather than waiting. I asked if he found anything surprising during the surgery, anything that he didn't expect. He assured me he had not. As soon as a bed became available on the ward, I was moved out of the ICU and into a regular room. My room had widows that looked out over the San Francisco Bay. All was going well.

Receiving Such Loving Care

In my memory, those days in the hospital are bathed in golden light. Each time I was asked my pain level on a scale of one to ten, my report was zero. I didn't expect that. I also didn't expect my elevated mood. If you were to ask loved ones to describe me ordinarily, they might use words like *serious, thoughtful, intense,* but in the hospital I discovered "light-hearted Marilyn." It is not that I'm never light-hearted in my normal life. I find my way there, but it isn't my perpetual way of being. In the hospital, it was. I was uplifted, curious, adventurous, welcoming, and I continued to find humor in almost everything. Maybe I was just incredibly relieved to have this long-awaited surgery over, or maybe it was a side-effect of the Fentanyl. I don't know, but I was so very grateful.

One afternoon, a nurse marveled at how accepting I was of whatever they needed to do. "We come in and tell you it's time for your shot, and you just say okay, thank you. Usually we hear, *Oh no! Not already. Didn't you just do that?* You seem fine with whatever needs to happen. How are you managing that?" I don't remember how I answered that question at the time, but I think now that it was due to all my preparation. I had succeeded in welcoming my surgery, and now I was continuing to welcome whatever was required for my recovery. I felt nothing but gratitude for all the help that I was receiving.

They were taking such excellent care of me. More than once when the door to my room closed after a nurse had been in to see to me, I lay snuggled in my bed feeling grateful that my every need was being met. I was being treated with so much kindness, such caring. I wondered how they could do that, every one of them, every day, in every instance. How is that even possible? I was also so supported by my friends and family. They sat with me every day and into the evening, helping in whatever way they could. I felt so loved. What could be better for my healing?

I soon got used to the fact that teams of medical people came on rounds early every morning. There was the surgery team, the plastic surgery team, and the pain specialist. At first, I thought the head resident of the surgery team was a little full of himself. Later I thought maybe he was just uncomfortable connecting. The team of women behind him were always smiling and nodding their heads encouragingly. This was another thing that struck me funny. I soon found myself playing a little game. I was determined to connect with that resident and sure enough, he came out of his shell. One day, when he gave me an encouraging little pinch on my shoulder, I knew I had succeeded.

I didn't expect to see Dr. Adam as the days went on. I thought my care would be turned over to the hospitalists, but he stopped in every single day except one, and on that day, he called to check in. It was always such a surprise to see him come through my door. I can't really explain the complexity of feelings I had for this man and his gifts, both personally and professionally. His stopping by each day gave me a great feeling of warmth and safety. I felt deeply cared for. His continued support was vital to my healing.

A Smooth (Mostly) Path to Departure

My hospital stay became a series of milestones met, indicating that my body was stabilizing and finding its way back to normalcy. As I've said, very soon after I woke up, they had removed the respirator. I got out of bed and walked on the second day. I left the ICU after three days. Once in my room, the catheter was removed. Each day I took a step towards body normalcy. Eventually the feeding tube went, and I could start eating. I continued to have no pain, except some very manageable gas pain when my intestines were first getting used to real food.

Joanna was by my side when my first meal arrived. It came with a cover over the plate to keep it warm. In great anticipation, we lifted the lid, and there, in all its glory, sat a scoop of mashed potatoes. What a feast! Soon after I was eating food, my bowels started functioning like they were supposed to. This brought enormous celebration from everyone. I hadn't been so celebrated in that way since I was a tiny child, yet another thing that struck me as very funny. This was a huge milestone.

Dr. Adam told me that walking was the most important thing I could do, as that helped the body to get everything lined up again and moving. I dedicated myself to walking as often as possible. Someone had to go with me to wheel the tower I was connected to with all the tubes and hoses. The nurses were happy when friends and family could help with my walks, freeing them to spend time with others.

My weight and all that extra fluid made me feel like a 90-year-old with congestive heart failure. My doctors were not concerned and continued to assure me that the diuretics they were giving me, and my own body would handle this problem, but it was what bothered me the most. I had a walker at first and thought of my dear old parents more than once as I walked down the hospital corridors. I was more than a little breathless and tired quickly, but gradually increased the number of my walks, each day trying to do more than the day before. We kept track of my progress on a chart on the wall, just for encouragement. I was also supposed to be breathing into a device called a *spirometer* that measured the amount of air I was able to breathe in and out, to be sure I didn't get pneumonia. We kept track of that on the chart as well. When I was weighed, the scale showed the pounds were dropping off rapidly, five or six pounds a day. That seemed like magic. There were times when I was dieting over the years and would have loved to have the scale falling so. It was quite surreal.

When I finally felt like doing some art, this drawing arrived. I titled it *Fluid Be Gone*.

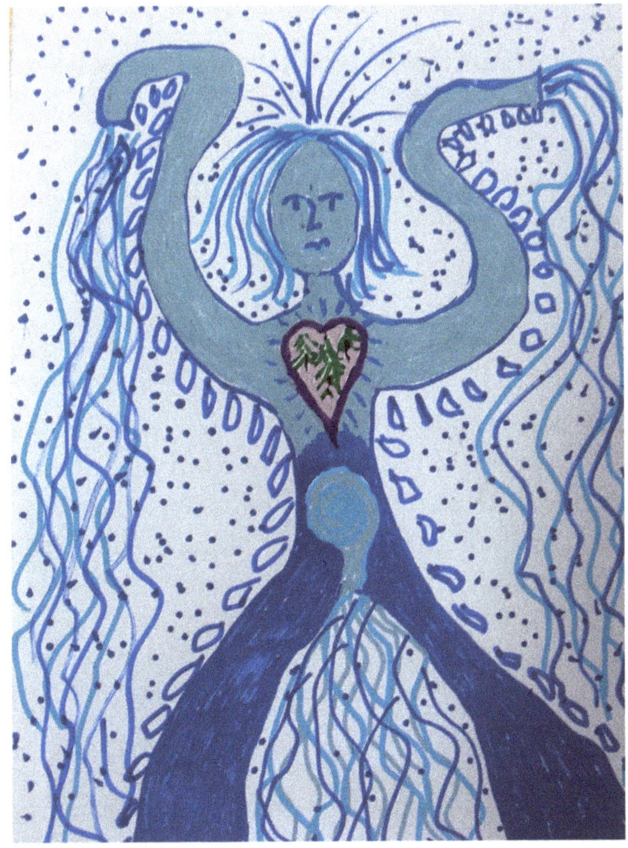

Fluid Be Gone

I did feel like an elephant with all that extra weight. Here my arms have turned into trunks, spraying the water away, my bladder pouring it out, my body perspiring it away. I so wanted for the fluid to leave my body any way it possibly could. In my heart, I drew my forest home, reminding me that it was there, waiting for me to return.

On the fifth day, they reduced the level of fentanyl coming into my epidural, and on the sixth day they stopped it altogether. It was time to make a bridge to oral medication for pain control. I was hesitant about taking oral opioids, but I didn't want to be naïve about pain, so I took the Oxycodone when they gave it to me. I entertained the nurse with my careful description of the affect. At first, I felt my head get very big and expansive. Then I felt like someone had put a heavy blanket on me. I became very, very tired. I could see that if I were a very anxious person, this might calm my mind, but my mind was already peaceful. My own sense of calm was deeper down in my body, not in my mind. I liked my own kind of calm better than this. This felt like suppression rather than peace.

Still, I was not experiencing any pain. Six hours later, when it was time for my second dose of Oxycodone, the nurse said I could try just taking Tylenol instead, which I did. Still no pain. I was so very lucky. On the second day of taking only Tylenol, the nurse said to me, "If you haven't experienced pain by now, you are not going to have surgical pain." I only took Tylenol from there on out.

One morning before the arrival of my family during visiting hours, I drew this picture.

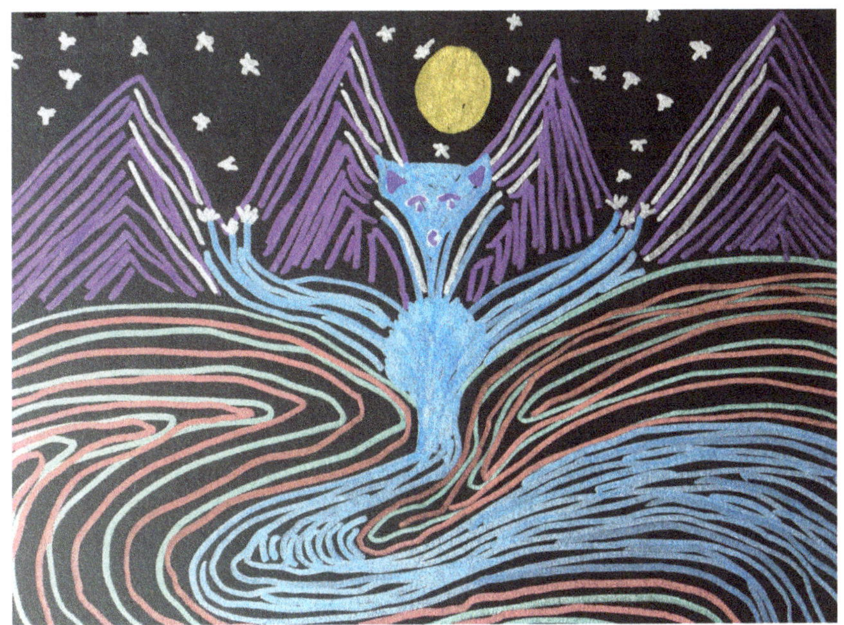

Fox Dreams

I was happy to have energy to do art and was just playing without having any particular intention. It began as a landscape, but then as the rivers flowed out of the mountain valleys, they joined together. I saw the water as a flowing figure. I gave it a head that turned out looking like a fox's head. I thought of my fox dream and its comment on my earlier surgery. Here I was, having been through surgery again. My psyche was still connecting the fox with the wounding from the incision of surgery. This fox seemed powerful and triumphant. I felt triumphant. I hoped this picture boded well for the further success of my treatment.

Darker Moments

While I hold my stay in the hospital with such positivity, I know there were darker moments. The afternoon they took my catheter out, I found I couldn't pee on my own. It was actually comical, how hard I tried. The dark part was that if I couldn't urinate within a few hours, they would have to put the catheter back in.

The last time I had visited my little grandson he was learning to use the potty. There were long sits there with his parents, while stories were read and songs were sung. Now, here I was sitting on the toilet. I tried to relax all those muscles, but nothing happened. I breathed deeply. I meditated. I turned the water on in the sink, thinking the sound of running water might help. I played watery sound effects on my iPhone. Finally, I even sang a little song, encouraging myself to let it flow, but all to no avail.

Having the catheter put back in was not a pleasant process, but three nurses lovingly labored, one holding a flashlight, one assisting and one putting it in. There was such celebration and relief when they succeeded. I was experiencing it all directly, but there was also a piece of me standing back and witnessing it as it was happening. As I looked down seeing those women trying to help me, I felt I was part of an age-old practice of women helping women, and my gratitude poured forth once again.

Another dark moment happened when the physician's assistant came in late in the day and told me that I had spiked a small fever. They wanted to get right on it if there might be a problem, so they ordered several tests. I became concerned. Everything about my recovery had gone so smoothly. The day before Dr. Adam had said he was pleased with how I was doing but did warn me that we weren't out of the woods yet. I didn't know when all those complications he had informed me about might show their ugly heads. That afternoon when I spiked the fever, I was worried that my good luck might be leaving me. Dr. Adam happened to arrive just a short time later. In his characteristic laid-back manner, he asked what was happening and then told me he wasn't concerned. In fact, he thought

I might be ready to go home in the next couple of days. *What?* That was a surprise. I was only on day seven of an expected fourteen day stay.

The fever turned out to be nothing. They thought I was going to go home on day eight after my surgery, but my oxygen levels weren't quite right. My night had not gone well. I had wild, frightening dreams and had awakened that morning with chest pressure. It was decided that I should stay an extra night. I wonder now if that wild night was caused by the fentanyl clearing from my nervous system, my body returning to being vulnerable to fear. I'm not sure Dr. Adam would agree that my altered state had to do with the medication, but I was feeling a level of anxiety that was unfamiliar to me.

My son Erik had been given a heads-up about my early departure and had driven from Utah to pick me up and take me home. He stayed with me in the hospital that extra day. The next day I was released. Dressing to leave the hospital, I felt like Cinderella's stepsisters as my feet were so swollen, they wouldn't fit into my shoes. I was wheeled out the door in my stocking feet and set free. I was nervous about the long drive, but I couldn't wait to get home.

Chapter 11

Home is Where We Go to Heal

"I hear your son is going to pick you up and stay with you for a bit," commented the hospital physical therapist when she came to evaluate me and approve my discharge plan. "I assumed I would be discharging you to a care facility. You are lucky."

Boy, did I know it. I live alone. The hospital could not have sent me home by myself to an empty house. If my son hadn't been coming to take care of me, they would have sent me to a nursing home. While that may have been fine, I was indeed lucky to have been discharged into the care of my loving son.

When they wheeled me out the door, Erik was waiting there in the loading area to drive me home. He would be with me for a week, then Gabe was coming, and then Eli. I would have one of my sons with me continuously until just after Christmas. I had never depended on them for that kind of steady support, until this illness came into my life. I knew my sons loved me, but their ready offers to come from afar to help made their love visible in a whole new way.

It was a bright sunny December morning as we drove through the streets of San Francisco and headed north across the Golden Gate Bridge. The world seemed a very busy place after my week in the hospital. I was a bit dazed, as if I weren't really a part of it all, but there I was, speeding down the freeway just like everyone else.

What was all this urgency? I wondered. *What's with the rush?*

We stopped at a supermarket to get something for lunch. Because our drive was already so long, we didn't want to extend it any more than necessary by stopping at a restaurant. I stayed in the car while Erik went into the store to search out food items I was allowed to eat. As I sat there waiting for him to return, I watched all the people walking in and out of the store. They walked fast and without effort, no towers with hoses and tubes were in sight. They all seemed to be moving through their world effortlessly, as we do when we are healthy, and mostly take our mobility for granted. I wondered if even one of them was grateful, in that moment, for their ability to move about so easily. I was humbled by my own vulnerability. I didn't want to forget my gratitude, but I could see how easily it could begin to slip away.

I came out of my reverie when I realized it would be good for me to get out of the car and walk a bit to keep my circulation going. I stepped out onto the asphalt in my stocking feet, held on to the side of the car, circling it before I climbed back in. Erik soon returned with a bag full of goodies. A few more stretch breaks along the way, and we made it home in good time. I was amazed that I didn't need to fall into bed immediately. Sitting in a chair in my kitchen, I visited with Erik while he made us some dinner. After all my preparation and all I had gone through, here I was in my life after surgery.

A New Level of Vulnerability

When I left the hospital, Dr. Adam said to me, "Hospitals are where we save lives. Home is where we go to heal." I had looked so forward to coming home, but once there, I was overwhelmed. My beautiful home in the forest seemed cavernous and cold. I felt very small in it. I was receiving much loving care, but I felt more vulnerable than I ever remembered feeling before. It didn't help that my nights were fractured and jarring. I repeatedly woke myself up shouting and fending off shadowy figures by punching the air with my fists, literally. Once I hit myself in the face while dreaming I was feeding myself forbidden food. The low residue diet was hard to deal with. There were so many things I couldn't eat. I was allowed ice cream which was the high point of each day.

In those early days, I was lost in the world of the physical, doing only what my physical body demanded from moment to moment, just the basics, eating, sleeping, letting bodily processes try to regain some balance. Energy was scarce to nonexistent. I lived in my recliner in the living room during the day, napping off and on, sleeping much more than I had at the hospital. When I would try to come to the table to eat, I had to brace my arms on the table to keep myself sitting in that hard wooden chair long enough to eat my meal. The elation I felt in the hospital was gone. My life just felt jagged.

Before surgery, Dr. Adam had said that a major surgery makes you feel like you have been run over by a truck. While I didn't feel that way in the hospital, it was an apt description now that I was home. I don't think I have ever experienced having no energy at all. It was hard to find motivation to do anything, even to get up and walk to the bathroom. Organizing for my first shower, I asked Erik to help me get some clean clothes together. He reached into my underwear drawer and pulled out a pair of bubble gum pink panties. I looked at them and said, "No, not those. Isn't there a different color in there?" It was as if I couldn't even imagine putting that bright color on my body, too much energy to bear. We both laughed.

Above all, I was supposed to keep walking, but it was hard to make myself do it. It was unusually cold outside with the forest holding all the moisture from recent rains. Even short walks were too much and left me panting. My poor body was still working hard to clear all that fluid. The weight was still falling off me by several pounds a day. I realize now that perhaps I should have just done laps around the inside of my house, but I yearned to be outdoors. However, walking in the forest didn't turn out as I had expected.

One day early in that first week home, I was holding onto Erik's arm as we walked down the path to my house on a late afternoon walk. I was surprised when the forest surrounding me felt ominous, like the trees were leaning toward me with bad intention. The forest has always been deeply nurturing to me. While I may have been leery of wild creatures in the forest, never once, in all my years, had I experienced the trees in the forest as threatening. What was happening to me? Erik was as surprised as I was when I mentioned it to him. Sometime later I did this drawing to express something of what I was experiencing in that moment.

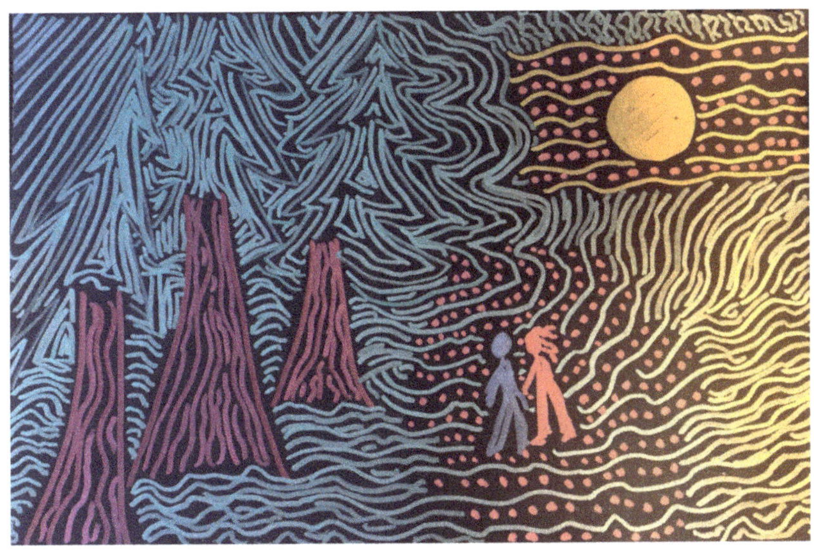

The Ominous Forest

The drawing looked psychedelic to me. It spoke loudly about the alive energy of the forest, like maybe I was perceiving it in some new way. When I thought about the ominous quality of the experience, I realized that I felt so vulnerable and was so deep into my physical experience that my animal body may have been perceiving threat that I wouldn't ordinarily have experienced. Thankfully, this only happened one time, but it was impactful. Sometime later when my twenty-something niece heard my story of the warm, golden glow of my hospital stay and then this spooky experience with the forest around my home, she was certain that I was in withdrawal from the fentanyl. I asked Dr. Adam about that, but he didn't agree, explaining once again that the fentanyl they had given me went into my nervous system, not into my blood stream.

Those are just a few of the iconic moments that stand out to me now, but much of how it was in those early days at home is a blur to me. What I will never forget is how lucky I was to have my loving sons and a circle of friends helping me through this challenging time.

Living in the Trauma

When recovering from an illness, I was used to feeling a little better each day, but that's not how it worked in the first couple of months after my surgery. Life was like a roller coaster, full of ups and downs, some days good and some days not so good. I measured progress from week to week rather than from day to day. I knew I was one of the lucky ones. None of the complications that Dr. Adam had warned me about had happened. For that I was grateful, but I was subdued. With hindsight, I realize I had been traumatized and was still living in the trauma. Coming to terms with that fact was a slow, gradual process and took months. At the time I was too much in the middle of it all, just moving from one moment to the next to get through my day.

It was a *tour de force* to go back down to San Francisco for a check-up, two weeks after I had returned home. Gabriel was helping me during that time. We drove through pouring rain, arriving the night before to stay in a hotel for my early morning appointment. I wasn't sure that I could walk far enough to navigate my way in the hotel or at UCSF, but I managed. I got a good report from Dr. Adam. All was going well with my physical healing. He empathized with my struggle and talked again about the trauma of major surgery. I heard the word "trauma," but I was not yet connecting emotionally to what that meant for me. I was still *in* the trauma.

My appointment was on my birthday, December 14th. I turned 76 that day. Returning home that night, I found bouquets of flowers at my door and more inside on my table. There were gifts too, from friends wishing me a Happy Birthday. There was so much love coming my way as I moved through this time of struggle. Once again, I was aware that having so much support was a big part of my successful healing. Dr. Adam confirmed that again and again.

I had been in the hospital on Thanksgiving but not yet eating, so no turkey dinner for me. I celebrated that holiday by wishing all the nurses Happy Thanksgiving and thanking them for working that day. I was at home and Eli was helping me by the time Christmas rolled around. On Christmas morning, he made Aebleskiver, the little round Danish pancakes that were our family's traditional Christmas breakfast, but my heart was not in the holiday spirit.

I still felt far away from what was going on in the outer world. Each of my sons had taken me down to my beloved trail on the headlands to walk as I was able, but I was not out in the world any more than that. Celebrating the holidays in my usual way was not in the cards, but I was feeling well loved, and that was probably closer to the true meaning of the holiday season.

As the new year rolled around, I was on my own for the first time. Friends stepped in to shop, help cook, and anything else I needed. I was incredibly grateful for all the help. My daughter-in-law had sent me a puzzle to help me bide my time while I was healing. My energy was limited, but I sat, putting it together for as long as I could before heading for my recliner to rest once again. It didn't escape me that working that puzzle, step by step, was a perfect metaphor for how I was, piece by piece, putting my life back together at that time.

Friends were stopping by to visit or to help, but internally I felt I was off in my own universe as I rested and waited for healing to take place. I remember thinking at the time that my friends were coming from another world. They were helping me stay connected to the web of my life before surgery, a world I hoped to return to at some point in the future. I was not there yet.

Struggling to Find My New Self

As my energy slowly returned, I was inspired to return to art making. I did a series of drawings, working in a small format on black paper with iridescent pens. I could easily draw in my lap while resting in my recliner. I had been wanting to draw something about my experience with Erik and the forest that day. That was the first one I did, followed quickly by several others.

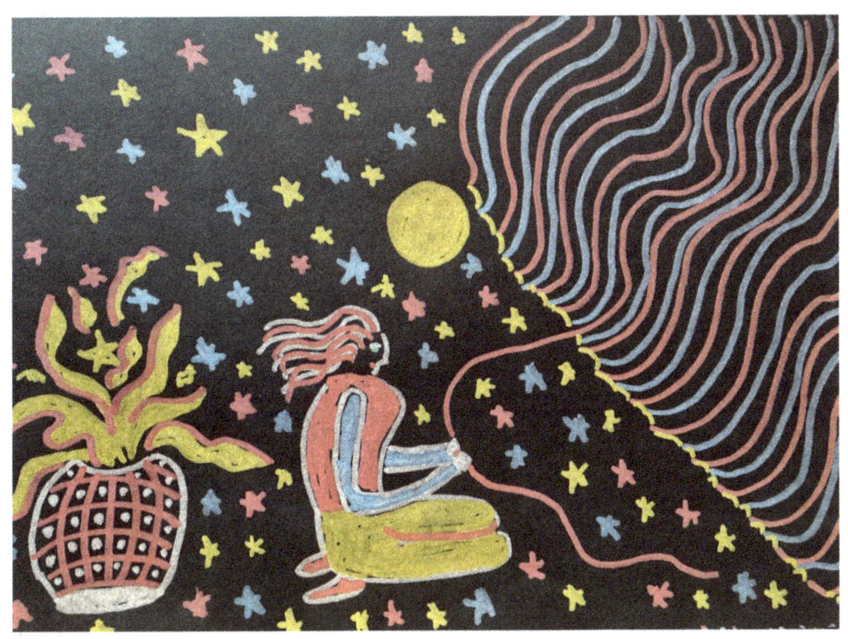

Holding the Thread of Life

When I drew *Holding the Thread of Life,* I was thinking about my friends' visits helping me stay connected to the web of my old life. Each visit was like holding a thread from that other world where all was normal. I was holding onto it with both hands as if I might just drift off into the universe if I didn't keep a grip on it. I didn't want to lose touch with that world, but I had to wonder, *Was there a normal life for me to return to?* The Marilyn I once knew was nowhere to be seen. There was someone there in that new body, a body that was missing so many parts now and bore a snake-like scar from pelvis to sternum. She walked, she talked, she was me, but she was not the me I once knew. She was unfocused, unformed, amorphous. She brought chaos and couldn't be counted on.

In my calmer moments, I remembered the butterfly coming out of a cocoon, a healing image that was following me. It helped me frame what I was experiencing. Looking again at my drawing, I saw it in a new way. I likened the universe I felt alone in to how the caterpillar might feel inside the cocoon, and all those wavy lines in the upper right of my drawing vaguely suggested a butterfly. Perhaps that thread I was holding onto was my attempt to bring to life my new manifestation. I had been through a transformative experience. As the butterfly, I was opening my eyes in a new world that I didn't yet have a handle on. Confusion reigned.

As weeks had turned into a month or more, I still felt pretty flattened by it all. Dr. Adam told me that in two months I would be feeling much more like myself. That felt doable when I first heard it, but two months lived day by day is actually a very long time.

In my drawing, entitled *Flattened*, I was expressing how weighted down I felt.

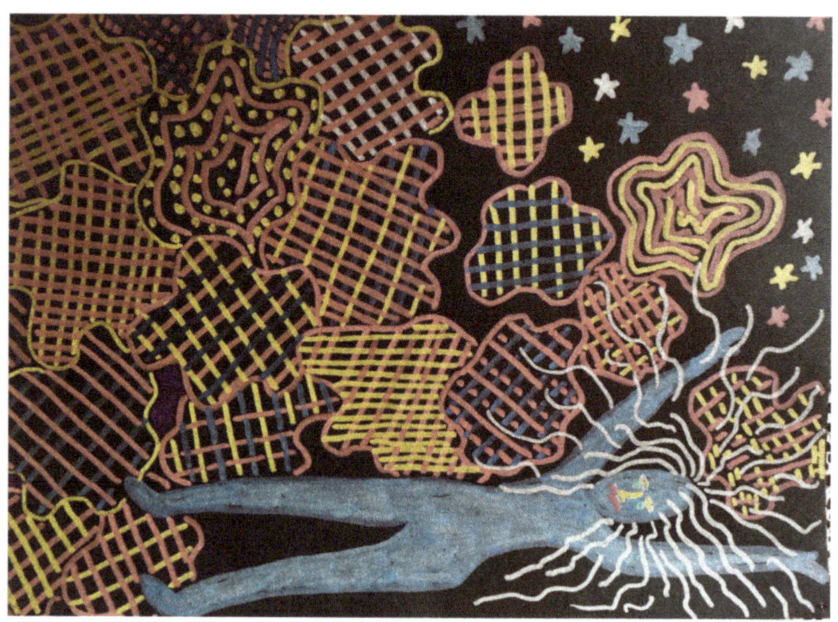

Flattened

It was as if I were trying to dig myself out of an avalanche of boulders. I found a crack where my arm reached out to freedom, but it was a narrow passage, not exactly an open birth canal. Also pictured here was my concern about my hair falling out. It wasn't falling out like hair falls out with systemic chemotherapy, but the chemotherapy in my abdomen had seeped into my tissue. It was supposed to do that, to bring healing. It had evidently done that enough to cause hair loss, which doesn't always happen. I found handfuls of it in my brush, and when I washed my hair, I feared I would just wash it all away. I hadn't expected this, and if I had, I wouldn't have thought it would be as upsetting as it was. I missed my full head of hair, as if some of my power was embodied there. That surprised me.

When two months after my surgery finally rolled around, there was a shift. For one thing, I was able to begin transitioning to a normal diet. A variety of fruit, vegetables, whole wheat bread, nuts and seeds could all return. I love food, and the low residue diet had been a real sacrifice on my part. I celebrated the return of each previously banished food in an almost ritualistic way, approaching with near reverence my first whole wheat bread, my first salad.

I was able to do most of what I needed to do to take care of myself but not effortlessly. I needed to rest often, even in the middle of preparing a meal. I still had to be careful about lifting due to my hernia repair, so friends were still of great help. I had been advised not to lift anything over five pounds. That was extremely limiting. I was feeling more like myself as Dr. Adam had promised I would, but if I was waiting for the old me to return, there was a problem because I still couldn't find her. That is when I began to be impatient with the time it was taking me to heal.

I had known that I wouldn't go through this experience without it changing me. The fact is, I was so preoccupied with what had happened to the old me that I was having trouble spotting the new me. So much of me was looking backward rather than forward. I was still trying to figure out how it happened that I had lain on the operating table for ten hours and survived, how I lived under the golden haze of the fentanyl for six days in the hospital, freeing me of all pain, how I had managed to struggle through as much of a recovery as I had. I was slogging through it all but with little perspective. I was lost in a mishmash of wonderment at how it was possible that my life had taken this crazy turn.

Where was I now?

Chapter 12

The Body Speaks

Ibecame increasingly impatient with the time it was taking to recover. I knew that wasn't useful, but I couldn't always control it. I was so much better than I had been, but I couldn't quite yet imagine picking up my life where I left off. Whatever power I felt before my surgery—the power I felt in my work, the power I felt in being a newly published author, the power I felt in my creative expression—now seemed an innocent illusion. What I had been through in the last year was incredibly humbling. If that power I had once felt had come from feeling healthy and invincible, it was long gone.

Where was my power now?

When I was caring for my elderly parents at the end of their lives, I found that when a crisis emerged, I did whatever was necessary to get us through it. It was only after everything had calmed down that my emotional response to the crisis finally had a chance to reveal itself. This same thing happened regarding my surgery. As I was able to live a more normal life, the emotions connected to the fact that I had been wounded by this whole experience began to dawn on me. I know it might seem strange that it didn't all happen at once, but it didn't for me. Yes, my rational mind completely understood that the wounding had happened in order to bring healing, but I was now having a growing awareness that no matter what the intention, I had still been traumatized.

Confronting Trauma

I shocked myself when one day, I realized with dismay, that my dear Dr. Adam had been the one who actually did this wounding I endured. He is the one who cut into my flesh! Even though I had given my permission in the deepest way I knew how, I was feeling the trauma of it now. For a brief moment, I wondered if it might be hard to see him again at my next appointment. How would I feel? This was not my best thinking. This was the voice of trauma speaking.

Perhaps Dr. Adam had given me permission to let these dark thoughts arise. I recalled what he had said to me, regarding dealing with pain after surgery: *We surgeons cause the pain. We need to help you do something about it afterwards.*

Physical pain was not my problem, but the trauma to my psyche was something real. I doubt that was addressed in medical school. Here I was again, with the curtain pulled away from all the usual conventions. In our conscious minds, we may understand and agree to surgery. I had prepared myself so carefully, but underneath it all, the body has its more direct, less conscious, literal way of seeing the situation. I recalled an old therapist telling me that arguing with the body is like arguing with a two-year-old. Nothing is rational!

If I've learned anything in life, I know I would not be who I am if I hadn't learned to listen to what my body had to say to me. I've learned to do that by paying attention to my subtle body energy, how it moves, where it is stuck. I tend to my emotions, acknowledging their contribution to my life. It is my body that dreams and talks to me in imagery, story, and emotion, rather than through any rational discourse. When I ask my rational mind to step aside, it's through the arts, through music, drawing and painting, and dance, that my body communicates with me. I have honed these practices over my adult life. I was grateful they were there, as now it seemed my body was ready to speak to me about my current trauma.

I trusted that process, even if it took me into dark corners. I didn't know if it was possible, but I'd had hints that my body knew more than my rational mind about what had happened to me during my surgery. I wish someone would study this. I've questioned doctors about it, especially anesthesiologists but to no avail. So I'm left wondering and paying attention to my own experience. As usual, making art helped me to explore.

I had spent two months healing physically, but the healing that was happening now was about something else. It was about acknowledging the wounding that had happened and then coming to terms with what it meant to me. Though I bore a scar on my skin, the surgery had taken place inside my abdomen. While I was in the hospital, I was shown a photograph of the tissue that had been removed during the surgery. It was all lined up and labeled. My friend and I referred to it playfully as the "meat market photo." That may have been an attempt to avoid thinking too seriously about the fact that it was my flesh that had been cut out of my body. Now I wanted to take a look, head on, at what had happened.

Turning to Art Again

When I started my drawing *The Wounded Healer*, I wanted to make marks representing all those wounds I had experienced inside my body. I wanted to put them on the outside of my body in my drawing. It was as if I wanted to externalize the wounding so I could see it. I wanted to make visible everything I had been through. These thoughts just arose in me one day, like something inside of me saying, *There is something you haven't been aware of. It is okay to open to it now. It is important for your full healing that you begin to look.*

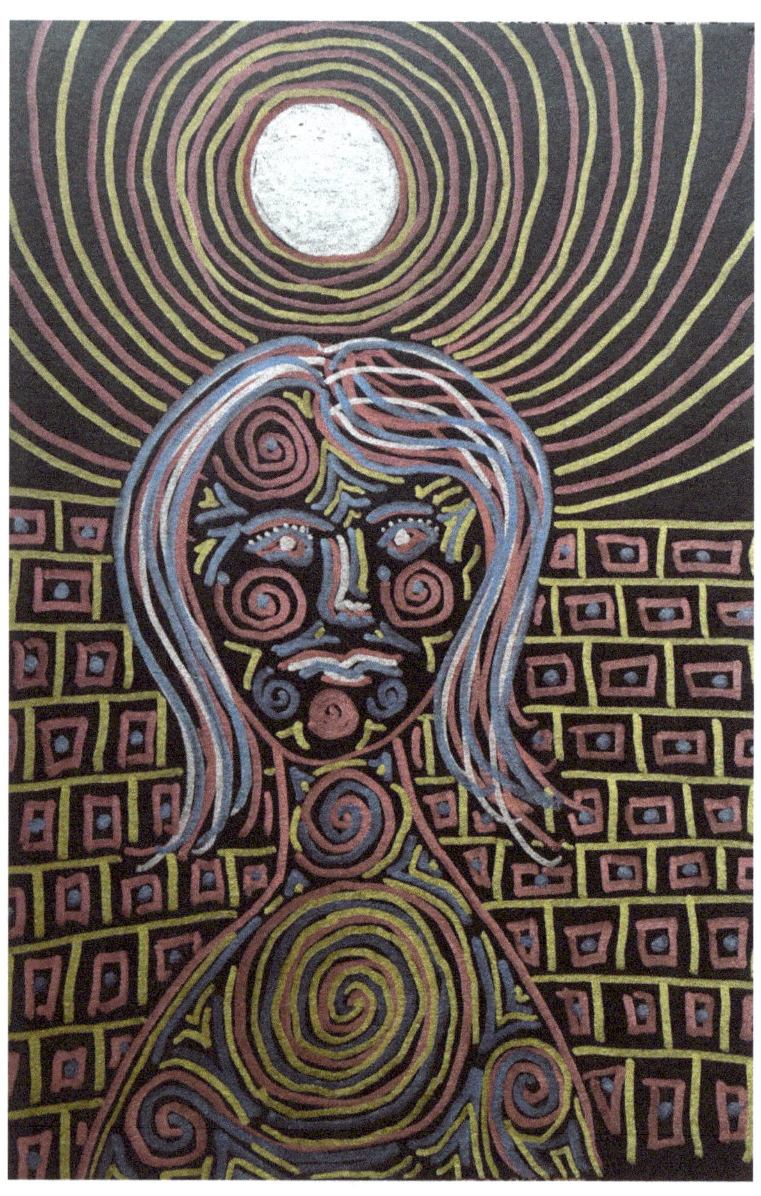

The Wounded Healer

I drew *The Wounded Healer* without thinking, almost like doodling, though I held my intention loosely in my mind. When I finished, I saw the primitive nature of what I had drawn. I couldn't help but see the background as a wall, perhaps the wall between my conscious and my unconscious mind. I had been living on the conscious side of that wall. This drawing was showing me what I couldn't see while I was so busy healing physically. It was showing me the unconscious side of the wall. As the light was returning to my life in that radiating circle above, it was illuminating that other side. I felt great compassion for myself when I looked at the drawing.

The primitive aspect of my drawing reminded me of shamanic cultures and suggested the spiritual nature of what I had experienced. I saw the Wounded Healer archetype represented there. That archetype holds the idea that our wounding is not for nothing, as through our own suffering we are given lessons and perspective that can help bring healing in our world. In this way, my drawing helped me place my personal suffering in a larger story and made it easier to hold.

This drawing was only the very beginning of dealing with the wounding I had experienced. It was the first inkling I had, a message from my body that something I wasn't conscious of had happened while I was under anesthesia for all those hours. My mind didn't know about it, but my body did know and was beginning to tell me something about it. Years ago, my therapist assured me that a healthy psyche takes care of us and only reveals from the unconscious what we are prepared to see. My dream mentor had told me something similar about what the unconscious reveals in dreams. When a dream brings up an issue, it is because the psyche is prepared to deal with it. I had come to trust that the same was true of art and what it might reveal.

My next drawing flowed naturally out of the feelings of woundedness expressed in my Wounded Healer drawing. In my life, I was back on my feet, but I was still very weary and tired of being weary. I wanted to draw something about that. I drew myself as a tree, but whereas before my limbs would have been lifting to the sky, they now felt weighted, cracked, and broken, unable to rise.

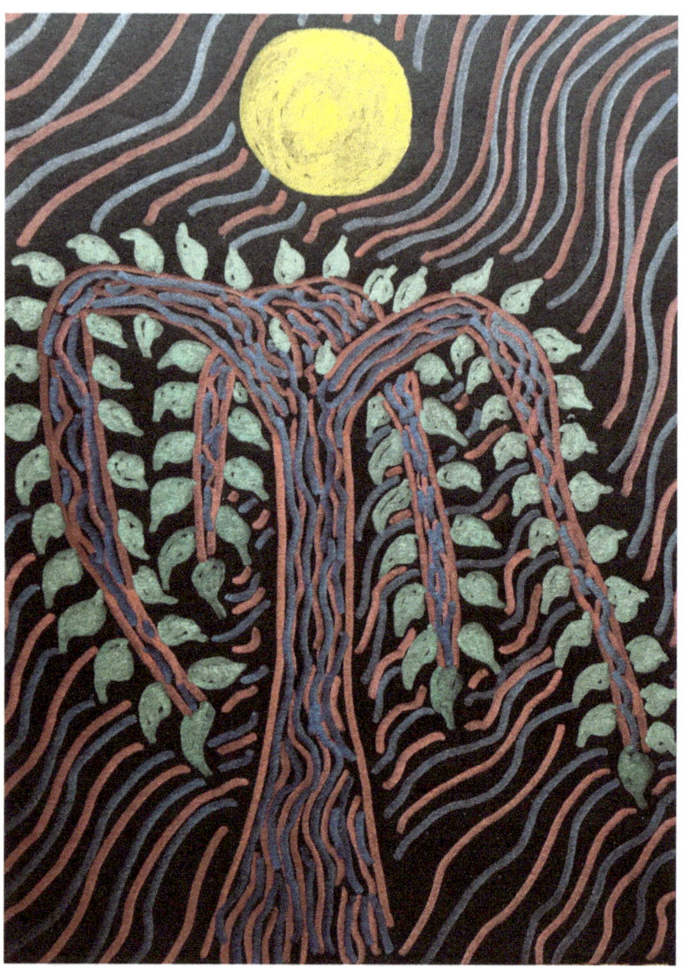

My Tree Self

When I finished, I titled the drawing *My Tree Self*. It looked more like a Weeping Willow tree than a tree with broken branches. It was as if I had risen but couldn't straighten up all the way yet. I felt great compassion for my weary self when I spent time with this drawing. My tears are usually easy to find, sometimes too easy, but I had not actually cried through my whole recovery time. Was this Weeping Willow telling me that I had been through a lot and survived? *Look, you have made it out from under those boulders. You were wounded, but you are standing. It's okay if you want to weep now.* I didn't cry, but perhaps my art was trying to gently reawaken that part of me.

As I lived with my drawing, I noticed something else. In the crotch of the tree where the branches leave the trunk, there are two leaves by themselves. When I stepped back, they looked like eyes and just below was a dark spot that could be a mouth. I did not plan this but couldn't help but notice. My conscious mind would not likely draw a face with such a cock-eyed expression, but there it was. I saw pain and struggle in the face of that tree being. The full moon watched over this scene, illuminating the struggle and allowing me to witness it. When I make art, even if I don't like to see what I've expressed, there is a sense of relief in taking my feelings and putting them outside of me and down onto the paper. Just that little bit of distance allows space for a bigger perspective.

Stepping further back and looking at the picture as a whole, I saw a magnificent being with the full moon for its head and the tree trunk as its body, the branches waving in the energetic field that the background is creating with all that movement. This drawing just kept giving me a bigger and bigger picture of the forces I was trying to navigate, from the personal to the transpersonal. I found some peace and acceptance of the moment in this very big perspective.

Coming Out on The Other Side

When Valentine's Day rolled around, I was nearing the three-month anniversary of my surgery. Things had greatly improved in the last few weeks. Maybe I really was getting this surgery behind me. I wanted to honor Valentine's Day with some art. I had been held in circles of love during this time of my recovery and wanted to express something about that. My inner voice told me I was through with black paper. I drew this next painting without thinking of anything but the opening of my heart to life once again.

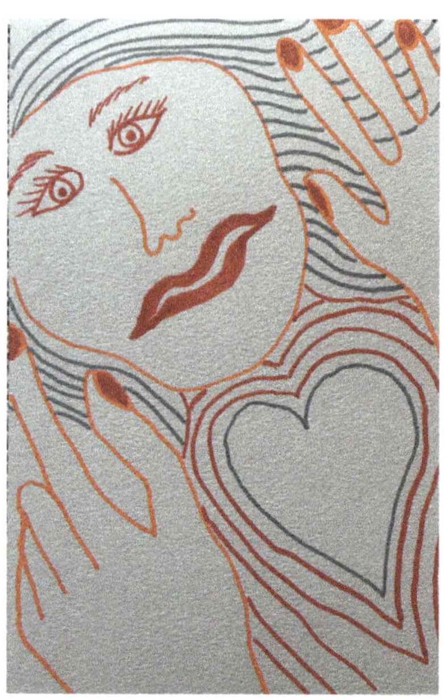

Circles of Love

I see such compassion in this face. She is someone who has known suffering and come through it with love. Was this me? I certainly hoped it was. Her hands seemed to be in a position of surrender. I was curious why her finger on one hand was pointing upwards. What was she saying? *Remember this,* or *Don't forget,* or *One more thing . . .* I had been so deeply embedded in my physical reality, in my body, perhaps now she was pointing to the heavens, reminding me of spirit. Perhaps she was saying all those things.

I wanted to write about all of this. I tried several times, but I couldn't yet find words. Creatively, all I wanted to do was make art. I continued to work in a small format, something I could hold in my lap, but now I craved white paper and color, intense color. When I drew this self-portrait, I wanted a close-up look at myself. I put that big sun behind me as a symbol of the light and energy that was returning to my life. It was like a new day was dawning. On this day, I was genuinely uplifted.

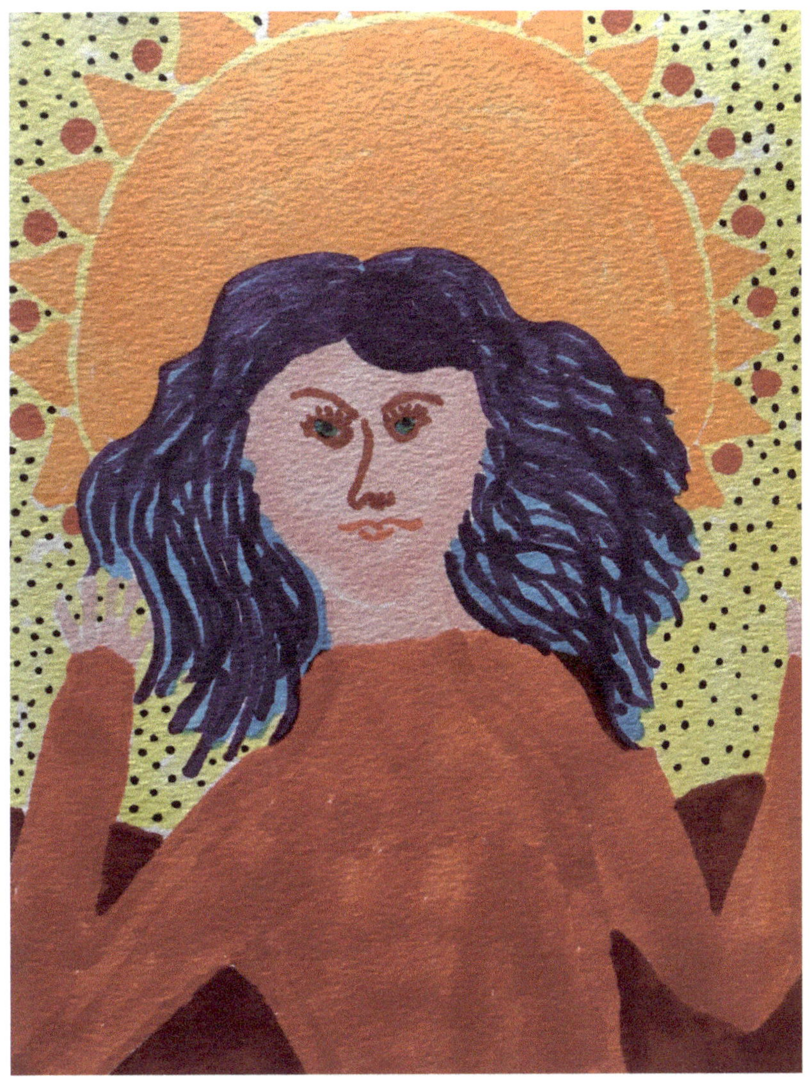

A Human Saint

When I finished my drawing, I was surprised to see that it looked like a religious icon. It continues to amaze me that even though I am not traditionally religious, Christian symbolism lives inside of me. Here it was emerging again. I entitled the drawing *A Human Saint*.

Did I feel myself a saint as I came through this crisis? I didn't know what that would mean. I shied away from feeling that special. I didn't grow up a Catholic. My church didn't have saints, so I didn't know that much about them. I did know that saints needed a miracle to prove their sainthood. I was entertained when the thought occurred to me that coming through my healing process, I had indeed performed a miracle. What miracle, one might ask? I am my body, and my body was healing itself. That was the miracle, but it didn't make me special. It just made me human. Was there sainthood in that? Maybe so, and if so, it belongs to all of us.

Whatever suffering I had endured, both mentally and physically, I was hopefully coming out the other side of, but it felt more like I was looking out a window, not quite yet ready to step out there. I felt vulnerable, like in a new skin, looking out onto an unfamiliar world. As I contemplated the end of my time in my healing cave, my hibernation, a question I started out with returned, but in a slightly different form.

Now What?

When I was deciding whether to have the surgery, my question was, *Am I being greedy in wanting more life?* What was stirring inside me now was the question, *Now what?* By having the surgery, I had challenged the forces that determine whether we live or die, and I had won, at least temporarily. It surprised me, but there was some discomfort in my victory. It would have been easy not to acknowledge that discomfort. I could have just been grateful to Dr. Adam and Western medicine, and called it good, but allowing that feeling to become conscious let me know something important. In deciding to be treated, I had taken my life into my own hands in a more powerful way than I ever had before.

We each wake up every morning and go about our lives. Whatever we think about life, whatever we do with our lives, so much of our activity runs on automatic pilot, even if we are contemplative and dedicate ourselves to finding meaning and purpose. Most of us don't wake up each morning saying, *I chose this day. I chose it at a cost. Now how am I going to use it?*

I had opted for the possibility of having more life. Now here I was on the cusp of stepping out into that more life. The question reverberating in the aftermath was, *What now? What was all that for? How do I want to use it?* I hoped to have given myself some precious time. That was all well and good, but there was also a darker voice with a more taunting tone, *What now? Whatever it is, it better be good. Come on, get on with it. Let's see what you've got. It better be worth it!* Oh dear! What a dilemma.

Then one night, I had a very physical dream.

I am in a powerful wrestling match with a man. He has invaded my space, and I am trying to get rid of him. We fight physically, and it goes on for a long time. I am aching and out of breath, using all my strength. I get myself in the right position to kick him hard in the shin, but when I play that forward in my mind, I realize that if I do that, I will experience the pain I inflict on him as if I am inflicting it on myself. I decide not to kick him.

I woke up physically exhausted, as if I had really been wrestling.

Initially, I saw this dream as wrestling with that dark voice inside me, the one shouting, *Let's see what you've got. It better be worth it!* It was the voice of the patriarchy challenging my worth once again. I didn't want that mean voice inside my head. In my dream, I'd fought back with everything I had. There was that message at the end, though. It was a slightly different reflection on that well-known bible verse, "Do unto others as you would have them do unto you." Transformed by the thought that we are all one, that message shifted to, "What we do to others, we also do to ourselves."

As I sat down to draw my dream, I thought about the biblical story of Jacob wrestling with the angel. It is a story that often comes up for me when I'm wrestling with spiritual matters. The image speaks so loudly of engaging intensely with spiritual questioning.

Though the guy in my dream was just a man, I gave him wings when I drew him, letting my dream image transform and find its way into a larger story.

In essence, I was allowing my personal image and my personal story to find its place in a mythological perspective. After all, myths are our collective dreams. They speak to the timeless questions about what it means to be human. I looked into it and found that the biblical story about Jacob has its roots in both ancient Greek and Egyptian mythology. When stories thread through time and culture, they become world stories. This frees them from their existence inside a particular time, culture, or belief system. In this way they offer us a peek into the depths of our human condition.

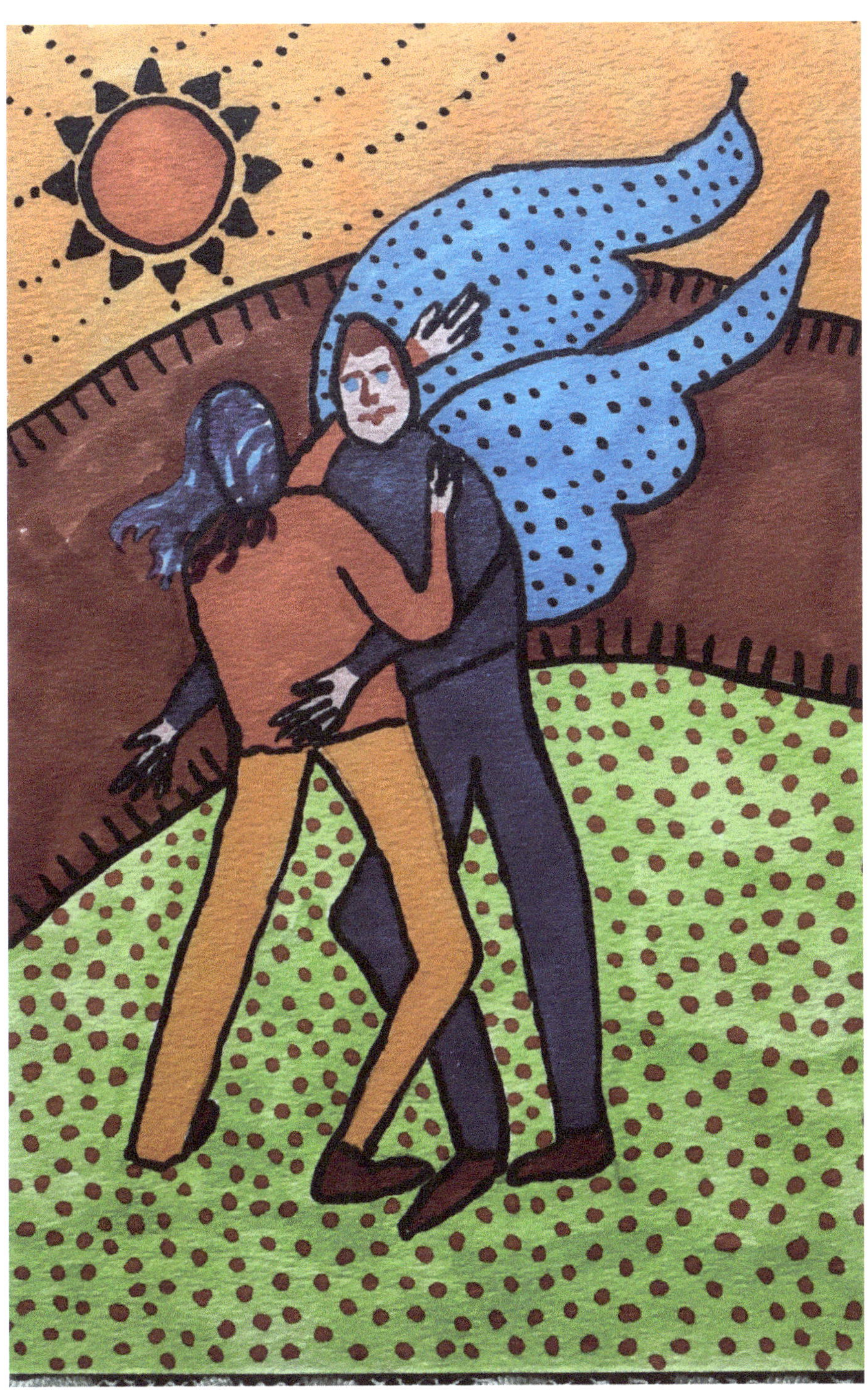

Wrestling with the Angel

I encountered the story of Jacob wrestling the angel in my childhood church. The image of the wrestling match stayed with me but little else about it did. I wanted to know more. Here is the gist of one version of that story: A man comes to wrestle with Jacob. They struggle all night long, and only when day begins to break does the man realize he is not going to prevail. The man wounds Jacob in the hip and then asks to be released. Jacob refuses unless the man, now revealed to be an angel, will bless him. When he receives his blessing, Jacob realizes that he has been wrestling with God. He names the place where this took place *Penuel*, which means The Face of God. His statement in one version of the Bible is: *For I have seen God face to face, and yet my life has been delivered.* It seemed like that was my condition as well.

I felt that in a way, I had entered this biblical story. In my dream I had wrestled with a man. In my art I had given the man wings bringing a spiritual perspective. My concern at the time was that I had wrestled with the forces in charge of whether I live or die. I had struggled, and I had been wounded. I had come face to face with a powerful force that I had not confronted before. I don't call that force God, even though I know it would be easier to have a name for it. I can't name it, but I understood that I had come into deeper relation with it. What would I make of that confrontation?

In my drawing, *Wrestling with the Angel*, it looks more like we are dancing than wrestling. The hands in the drawing aren't grasping. It is as if there had been a momentary embrace. Now life was going on. How would my life be different dancing with the knowledge I'd gained in that encounter?

In another painting from that same time, one I entitled *Remember This*, I am confronting death pictured here by a skeleton under the eclipsed sun. I am a little off to the side, as if this time I can walk right on by.

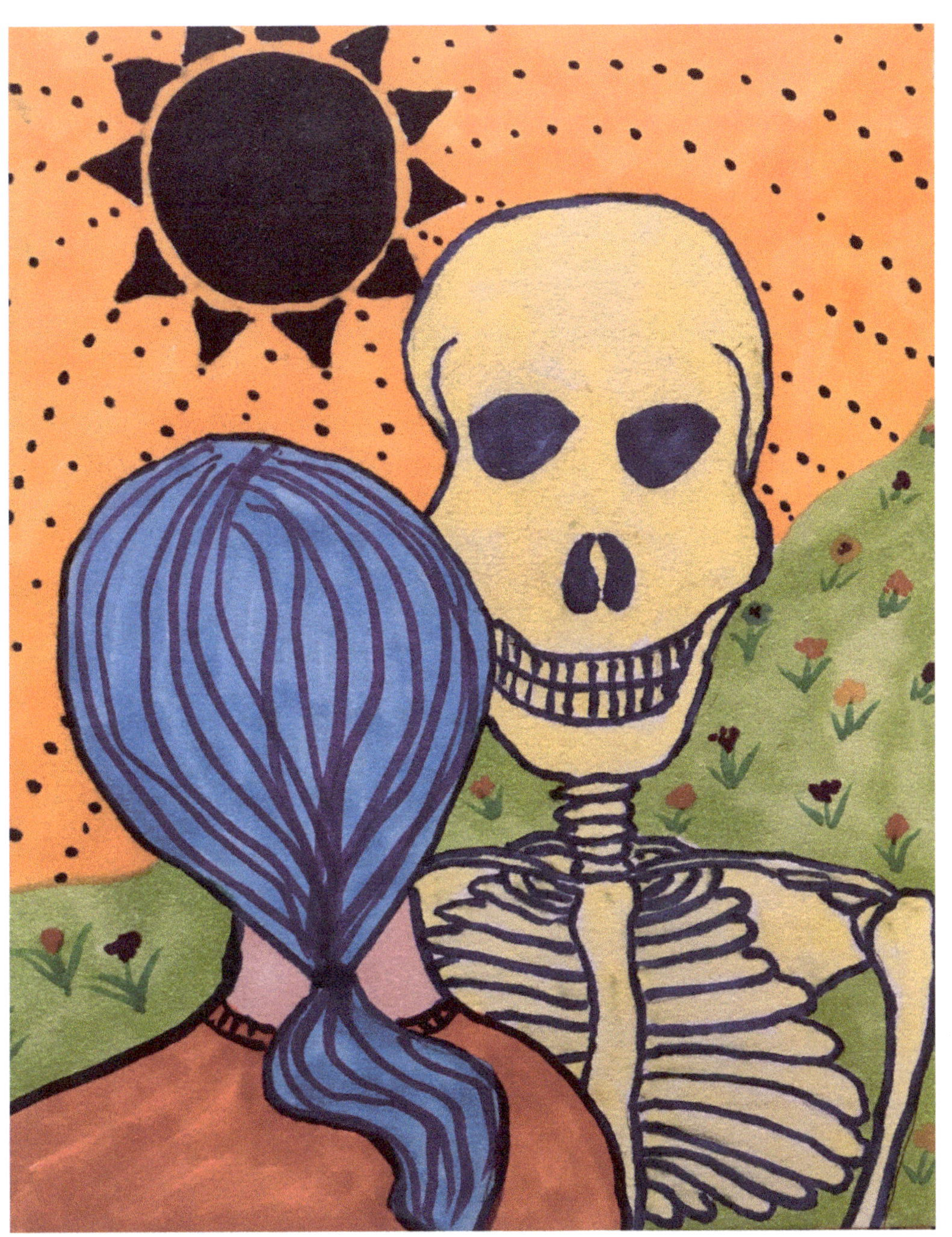

Remember This

I thought again of my drawing where that woman's finger pointed upward, perhaps saying, "Remember this." It seemed like my art was showing me what she was referring to. I wanted to remember this confrontation with death. I wanted to let it change me.

Life was moving on. I was ready to partake in more of my old life, but it wasn't easy to step back in. My natural introversion was well supported being home during my healing time, letting the world come to me rather than stepping back out into it. It felt like time to bring back the part of me that was more outgoing. On the day I was going to rejoin my women's group, I did this drawing which I titled *My Purple Heart.*

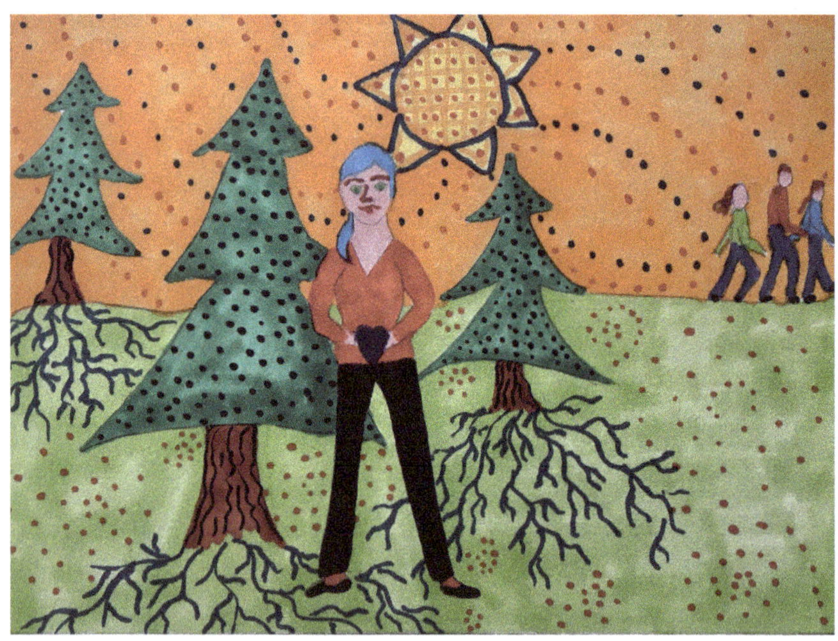

My Purple Heart

Here I am ready to step back out of my forest home and join my friends. I am standing. I am rooted like the trees around me. I'm holding a heart over my abdomen. I wanted to color my shirt red, so I couldn't paint that heart red, or it would be invisible. I chose purple without thinking. Then I realized I had given myself a purple heart, an honor given to the wounded in our military.

In my next drawing, I saw myself walking on my healing path. I even look energetic. There was still more to be healed, but I had come a long way. The path ahead was uphill, but things were taking shape. I was standing, even walking now, stepping out. The river of life was flowing there beside me. I was walking through an alive and vibrant world. On this day, I was optimistic. Things were looking up.

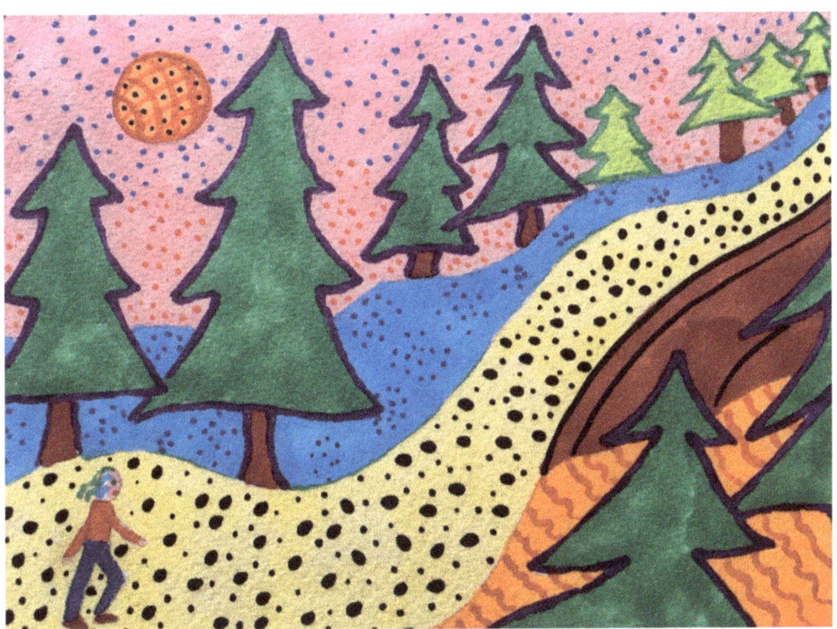

My Healing Path

Chapter 13:

Come On Come On:
The Future Beckons

When I was preparing for surgery, it had surprised me that I didn't use battle imagery in thinking of my upcoming procedure. It became clear, however, that I was battling both physically and mentally in order to recover from it all.

As my next appointment with Dr. Adam approached, I was getting nervous. My appointment was on March 10th, not quite four months after my surgery. All seemed to be going well. I wasn't expecting bad news, but after all I had gone through, it would feel terrible if that were to happen. I let that thought go, not wanting to focus on it.

As I began preparing for my appointment, I wanted to address the question, *What are my concerns now?* I did a drawing that I titled *Healing Body, Mind, and Soul* three months after my surgery. It felt like a snapshot in time, expressing how much I had healed but allowing my concerns to make themselves visible.

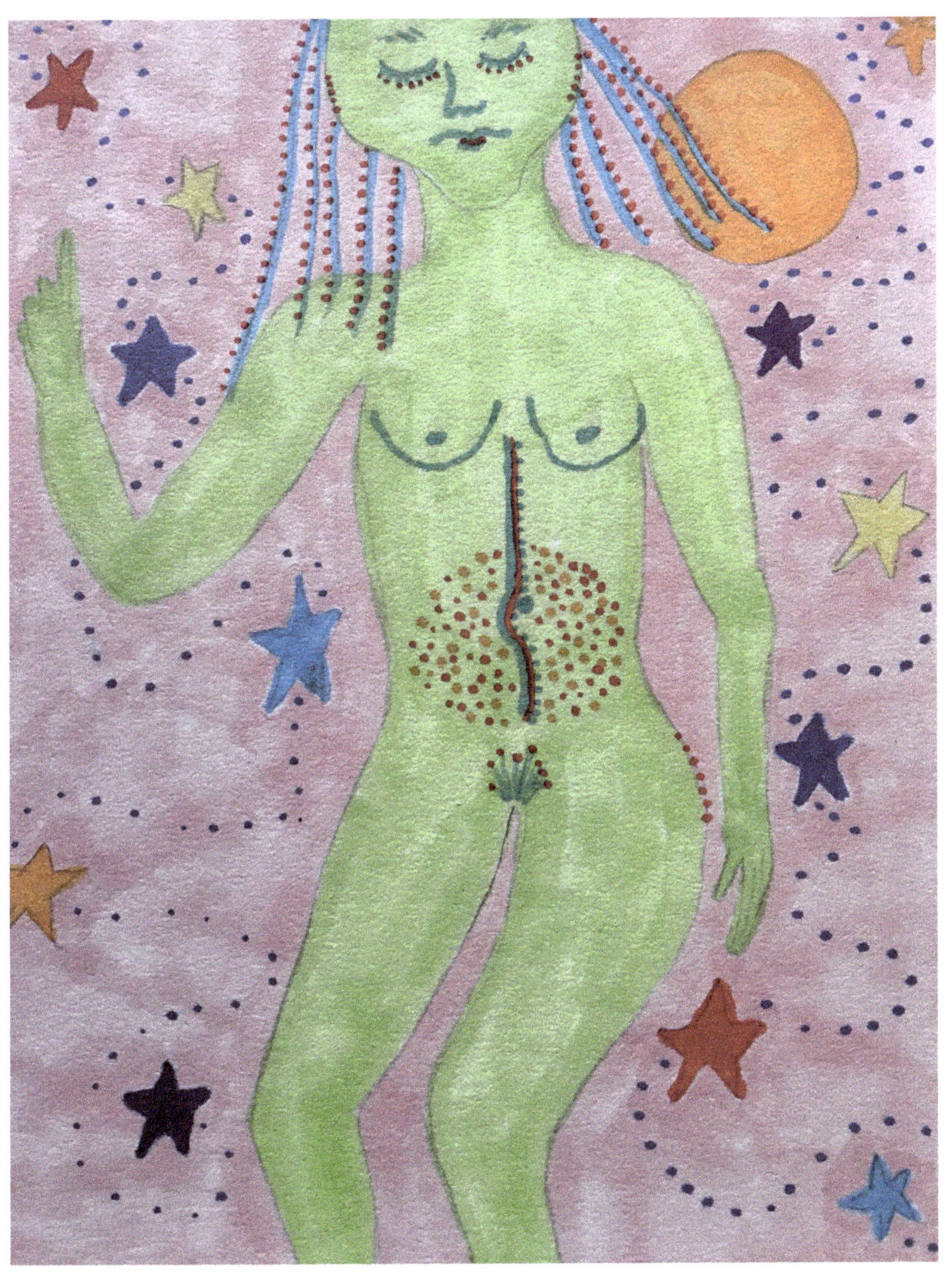

Healing Body, Mind and Soul

I loved the peace I felt while making this drawing. There was a marked difference from how I had felt making my previous pieces. I selected green for the woman, not knowing why, and then I painted the background where nighttime stars were visible in the light of day. At the very end, I placed the little red dots on her body, indicating places of concern. When I finished the drawing, I saw the green woman as me, green with healing, like the new grass in the springtime meadow of my forest home. The nighttime stars were a reminder of the darkness I had passed through on the way to this new dawn. The red dots indicated my remaining physical concerns, but the picture itself showed those concerns small in the scheme of things. I felt this drawing was a spiritual self-portrait, letting me know that on that level I was finding balance.

I did want to discuss the concerns pictured there with Dr. Adam. I also needed to hear from him about my future. I had struggled with that part, questioning what I wanted to know about it and how I could best hold that in my mind. I didn't know how to frame the question so the answer I received would promote my best chance to move forward with peace of mind.

As the day of my appointment neared, I became increasingly anxious. I had joked with a friend that I thought I was having PTSD symptoms when I thought about going back to the UCSF hospital. Rationally, that didn't make sense to me—I really was joking.

Thinking about all of this, I sat down to make art. An image of a cat curled up popped into my mind. I had been playing with tempera sticks on larger format paper and decided to go ahead and paint the cat. I laughed out loud when I saw how it turned out. It certainly looked like a scared cat to me, a *Scaredy Cat* indeed, which is the title I gave to this piece.

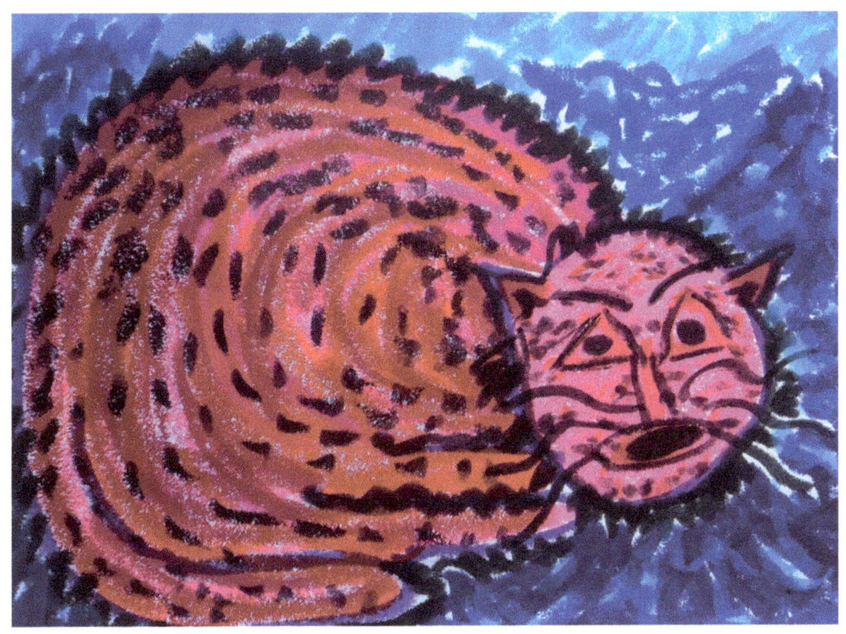

Scaredy Cat

I hadn't realized I was drawing a self-portrait, but there it was, whether I intended to draw that or not. I was afraid. The drawing didn't take away all my concern, but it did bring humor to the mix and that helped once again. I know that when you can rise above your troubles and laugh at yourself, it always helps to change your perspective. This Scaredy Cat did just that for me.

I asked my friend Joanna if once again she could come to my appointment with me. We had to spend the night in San Francisco and were going to be staying at the very same hotel where I had prepped the day before surgery. Returning now to the hotel, I didn't want to think about that very difficult day, but my body remembered it all, and when I woke up the morning of my appointment, I felt nauseous.

Rivers of Tears

I was scheduled to have an early morning CT scan before I saw Dr. Adam. It was not a good day in the radiology department. Perhaps those in charge were exhausted by the demands of the pandemic. I'm sure they weren't bad people, but that day it seemed like they were on automatic. I felt they treated me like a piece of meat that just needed to be run through their machine.

I had made the mistake of forgetting not to wear metal. The zipper on my jeans and the rhinestones on my shirt couldn't enter the machine. I wasn't offered a chance to change into a gown, so pants down around my ankles, blouse pulled up just beneath my breasts and arms stretched out over my head, I was rolled into the scanner. There was a longer than usual pause between scans, and my arms were in searing pain from being left in that position for such a long time. The technicians and nurses were in the room behind me chatting when I tried to get their attention. Tears brimmed and spilled over as I shouted "Hello?" louder and louder and louder. I was just about to switch to "Help!" when one finally emerged and asked if I was talking to them. I don't know who he thought I was talking to—they were the only people there. When he came over to see what was wrong and saw my tears, he became very solicitous and helped me get comfortable, and we finished the scan.

I knew that what had happened wasn't the end of the world, but when I left there, I couldn't stop my tears. It was as if the message, *It's okay if you want to weep now*, the one I'd gotten from my *Tree Self* drawing, had finally fully awakened inside of me. I sat in the car recounting my sad story to my friend. My tears flowed freely as I felt the humiliation of my pants down around my ankles, my blouse barely covering my breasts, their inattentiveness, my discomfort, their abandonment.

As waves of tears rose and fell, I began to realize that all this upset wasn't just about my difficult experience with the scan. All the tears I hadn't cried as I soldiered through these months after

my surgery were pouring out now. I was vulnerable, and returning to this physical place where my traumatic experience had
happened had broken a dam. I knew then that my anxiety and my
joking about PTSD may have had more relevance than I knew.

When I calmed down, I took a deep breath and sighed.
There was more to the day, and I didn't want to arrive in Dr.
Adam's office with red eyes and tear-stained cheeks. We went
to the cafeteria to get some breakfast. As I reflected, I realized
that I was a participant in what went wrong at my CT scan. In
my anxiety about the day, I had forgotten to reach out to the
assisting staff, to help them see my humanness. That had been
so important to me throughout the year of being a patient.

My friend objected: "A skilled person with a nurturing spirit
would do that naturally!" she replied, insisting that they should
be doing the reaching out, not me. I suppose she was right, but
the fact is that someone needs to bring more humanity to the
exchange. Why not me the patient? I wanted to accept my full
responsibility in what went wrong. Maybe those helpers were
having a bad day, maybe they were overworked and burned
out. They are only human after all, as am I.

Through this whole year, I hadn't wanted to find myself as
the victim of a mechanized, production-oriented medical system. With my new vulnerability came a deep desire for human
connection, not just with my doctor but with everyone who
would be helping me. As with Dr. Adam, I wanted to rely on
people's expertise, but I wanted our shared humanity in the
forefront of our interaction. Otherwise, I feared it would be
far too easy to become a victim of the system. That wouldn't be
good for any of us. I didn't want to shirk my part of the responsibility to bring that connection I wanted and needed. I knew
that bringing my humanity and ability to connect to all who
served me would make a difference in our interaction.

During that CT scan, I saw what happens when I forget to
bring all of me into the shared experience. That day, in my
cloud of uncertainty, I had forgotten to even try. I wasn't happy

to have missed an opportunity. By the time I got to Dr. Adam's office, my blood pressure was sky high and needed to be taken twice before it fell back into a normal range.

Good News

I was genuinely happy to see Dr. Adam when he entered the exam room. The feeling seemed mutual. Here we were on the other side of surgery and down the road a bit. He had reviewed my CT scan and blood tests. Everything looked good. You would think that hearing the good news from him, that my surgery and treatment had done what it was supposed to do, would bring instant celebration, but I couldn't seem to let that news in all at once. My response was more muted.

I found myself breathing more deeply as I heard that the scan was clear, and the blood tests were back in the normal range. He told me that I could put this behind me now and move on. When I asked if I should be watching for any symptom of my problem returning, he responded adamantly: "No. I wouldn't do that. We will be monitoring you with tests and scans, and that is all that will be needed."

Hearing my impatience about the slowness of my healing, Dr. Adam had to remind me several times what a traumatic event my surgery had been, that so many things could have gone wrong but hadn't.

Addressing My Future

When I look back on that appointment, I can feel my discomfort. I was still kind of lost. I told Dr. Adam that I was in a fog and confided that most of me was still turned toward the past. Some of me was in the present, but almost none of me was looking to the future. I knew I needed to pivot but was finding it hard to do that. Inside, I wondered if I even had a future. My diagnosis had brought that possibility into question. Now, I had gone through all of this, but the rupture with my future hadn't yet mended. I know that Buddhism would tell me to forget about the future, all we really have is the present moment. I don't disagree, and I understand the power of the timeless "now," but as a woman living in the world, certain practical considerations require being involved with the life yet to come. I needed to address the question of my future in my appointment, but it was a subject I wanted to approach carefully, so as not to elicit a response that would be troubling to me.

I have deep respect for the porosity of my psyche. I know that I am easily swayed by suggestion. I had proved that to myself years ago when I gave birth to my third son, Eli. It was all the rage where I lived to have your babies at home. We felt birth was a natural process, so why not have it take place in your natural environment rather than the hospital? Because I had had both Erik and Gabriel early, my doctor told me I could have Eli at home any time after June 15th but not before. Eli was born at five minutes after midnight, on that very day, an event fitting my doctor's suggestion about what the limit might be. Similarly, were Dr. Adam to tell me the average number of years people live after a treatment like mine, I was afraid I might live into that prediction. I know that may sound superstitious, but it is how I felt. I had spent weeks wondering what I needed to know about my future, and how I could think about it in a way that would be best for me. I hadn't come up with an answer.

"We did all of this because of your future," Dr. Adam reminded me. Then, with his words, he conjured up a felt sense of the river of time and our relation to it. "Likely, if I were to bet, you are not going to die because of this condition. It's been a big shock. You are doing all of this and all of that, it's a big event, and then you recover from it. Now it is done, you paid for it, one time. Now . . . move on. It's all behind your back."

With an audible sigh of relief, I felt myself standing on the threshold of a doorway to my future that I hadn't been able to locate on my own. Dr. Adam was pointing the way, telling me I could return to all my normal activities. He checked my incision and pronounced that it was well healed. He admired the handiwork of the plastic surgeon who had closed it with his skillful stitching.

On so many levels, I had breezed through this major event, especially considering my advanced age. Still, what I had gone through shouldn't be underestimated. It was a major, *major* trauma to my body. Dr. Adam didn't speak about the trauma to my psyche, but I felt the truth about his statement, for my body and my mind. I felt it in that very moment.

When I walked out of my appointment that day, I felt as if I were walking into a new world, one where breath came easier. As I walked out the door of the medical complex, I saw my future standing patiently there in front of me, as if it had just been waiting for me to notice it was there. If my awareness of the river of time had come to pause inside of me, I felt it flowing once again. I saw myself as if in a little boat, sailing down that river into my future. While I didn't feel completely recovered, I left with more gratitude for the healing that had taken place and with more hope that I would soon find my way to full recovery.

Taking Off My Patient Coat

Back home that next day, I found my step lighter on my morning walk. I walked farther and faster than I had been able to before. That is when the extent of the mental challenge of the recovery process became very concrete. It was my mindset that had been holding me back, not my body. In my imagination, as I walked, I felt myself burdened by the heavy coat I imagined I was wearing. I hadn't been aware of it before, but it felt like a part of me now. I supposed it had grown on me over this long year of being a patient. In the extreme vulnerability of these months of tests and surgeries, I must have felt like I needed its protection. Now it felt heavy and unnecessary. It was time to take it off.

When I got home, I made two drawings. I wanted to see what this heavy coat looked like. I titled the first one *My Patient Coat*

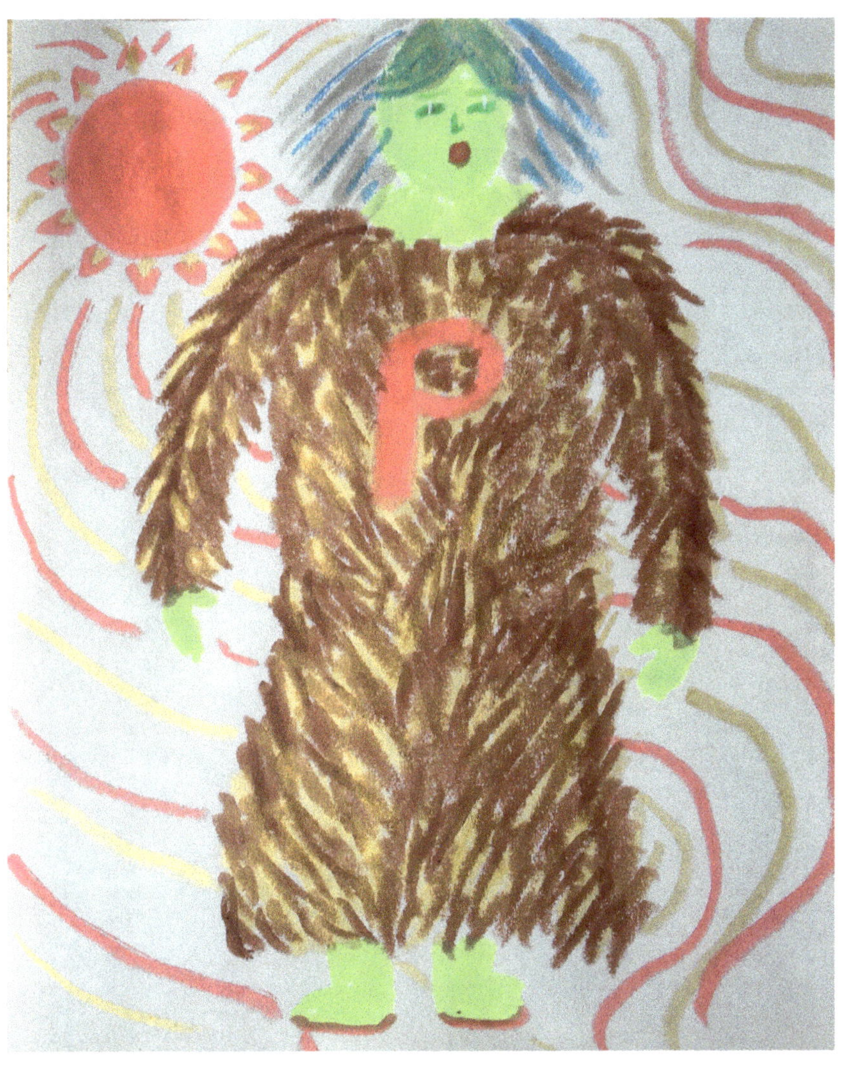

My Patient Coat

I was surprised to see so much fur. It suggested the animal nature of my experience, how ill health keeps the physical body at the top of awareness. The letter P, standing for *patient*, sits over my heart like the letter A in the tale of The Scarlet Letter, announcing my condition to all. Reflecting on my art as the days passed, I saw myself, spring green, under all that fur, and I became increasingly ready to take off my coat. *Who would I be without it?* I wondered. I wasn't at all certain.

My next drawing reveals me standing on my coat, floating down the river of time under a rosy, red sun. My scar, now looking like a snake running from pelvis to sternum, marks my journey as a healing one. I am balanced on my fur coat, representing my experience as a patient, looking ready to take on my new life, whatever it might bring. My finger points down as if to emphasis my place here on this beautiful earth.

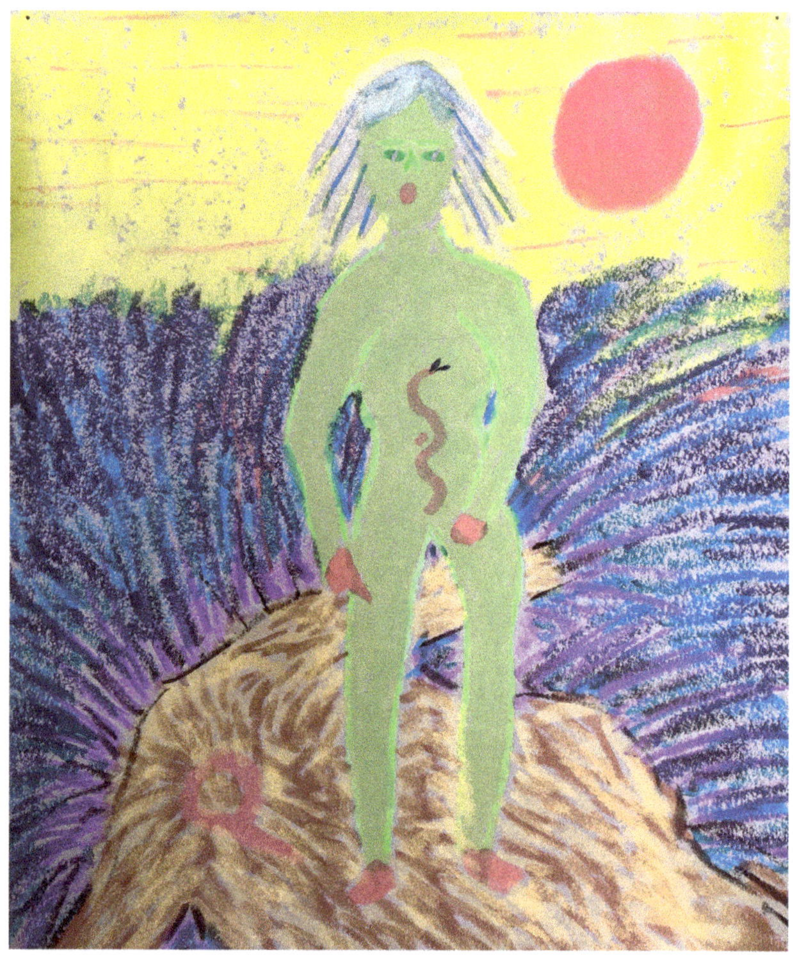

Floating on the River of Time

Another whole month went by. I was now over four months out from my surgery. As I walked into my living room one sunny April afternoon, I heard a voice in my head say, *I am a walking miracle!* A smile spread across my face, a little laugh followed. *What a thing to say!* I thought to myself, but the truth of it began to sink in and the fake humility faded away. In that moment, I truly felt like a walking miracle. That my body was able to heal from such a major trauma was indeed nothing short of a miracle.

The power of the human body to heal lives inside each one of us. It serves us over our entire lifetime in ways big and small. Mostly it goes unrecognized and unacknowledged as we take that healing power for granted. *It is just what bodies do,* we think, if we think about it at all. On some level, the body's thrust for repair is so ordinary, and on another level completely extraordinary. That day in my living room, the blinders were removed from my eyes and the shield over my heart unlocked. For one extraordinary moment, I felt the full extent of what recovery means. In response, gratitude poured out of me with such force I wanted to fall to the earth and kiss the ground.

To proclaim that I am a walking miracle let me know that I was standing firmly at the other end on this healing journey. We don't recognize a miracle until it has happened, so I must have reached my destination. I had wanted to feel celebratory when Dr. Adam told me that the treatment had done what it was supposed to do, but I had more to integrate and accept before that could happen. I had to spin the experiences of the last year into one single thread to hold the truth revealing itself in that moment in my living room.

To spin that thread, I needed to remember the shock and the fear, the giving up and the soldiering through, my surrender to the process, and the support of so many. I had to embrace all the suffering and all the love in order to make that thread sparkle with the vitality of my healing journey. Feelings of joy, relief, and gratitude bubbled up from my depths, overwhelming all my defenses. I knew I was accepting the darkness and the blessed light of my healing journey, and for the first time, I wholeheartedly celebrated my recovery.

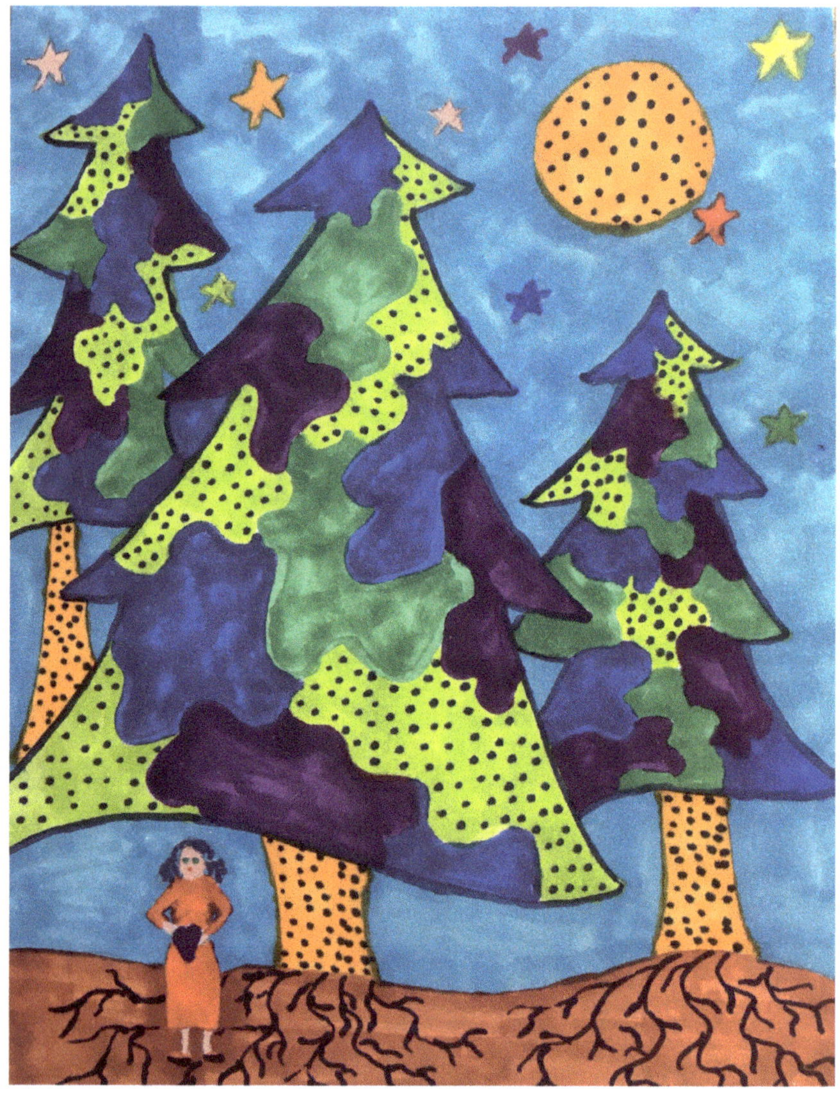

My Forest Home

Here I stand rooted back into my forest home, holding my purple heart. That wild energy of the forest I had experienced in the early days after I returned home is contained now, back inside of the trees. Night and day are pictured as one in the sky. I am at peace standing under the canopy of these forest guardians. Though small in the big picture of things, I stand tall. Life goes on.

Chapter 14

Don't Go Back to Sleep

While I celebrated my physical healing, I knew I was still quite fragile emotionally. So much had happened since I found that blood on the toilet tissue over a year ago. As April rolled around, and I was a little over four months into my recovery, I suspected that it would be a while before I integrated all I had learned from this experience.

I was aware of my fragility in many ways. I had been telling friends that I was through with being a patient. I was extra careful regarding my health, even as others were relaxing into new possibilities with Covid waning. I continued wearing my mask indoors in public. I avoided gatherings. I didn't want to get the flu. I didn't even want to catch a cold. I'd had it with anything even vaguely related to ill health and the vulnerability that comes along with it.

I had come through this surgery and was standing on my own two feet again, but like a little one just learning to walk, I was off balance. I knew that it wouldn't take much to topple me. And sure enough, it didn't.

A Complication Arises

On a Friday night, one week after April Fool's Day, my body had another surprise for me. When I got up to use the bathroom, I felt a burning pain in my left leg, just to the side of my knee. It was still there in the morning, and when I looked, I found a big red swollen area around a varicose vein. I figured it must be a blood clot and sure enough, when I saw my local doctor on Monday, my suspicion was confirmed. I had read online over the weekend that a clot in a varicose vein was not as serious as a clot in a deeper vein, but I didn't want a clot anywhere. While my doctor validated what I had read, she also let me know that because of my diagnosis and my recent surgery, it was something to take seriously. It couldn't just be ignored.

I suddenly felt the clot like a time bomb, which wasn't likely to go off but could, and if it did, my hard-earned future could explode with it. I recalled an article I had read before my surgery. It had reported that one in five people over sixty-five who have major abdominal surgery die within a year of the surgery. At the time, a friend had pointed out that I was in really good shape for my age and had taken very good care of myself over the years.

"Think of all the smokers and drinkers, people who've lived very hard lives," she told me. "You don't fit in that statistic." I never asked Dr. Adam about the report but funny how that seed had been planted inside me and popped up when my blood clot arrived. *Is this how it happens?* I wondered. *You make it through one thing, but something else is just waiting to take you down?* A morbid thought, I know, but it was the essence of the dark cloud the clot brought my way.

While more tests, doctor's appointments, and medications swirled throughout the weeks that followed, inside I found myself reorienting to my future or the lack of it once again. There had been a little voice in the back of my mind that knew my inner conversation about embracing my future was folly, but for a while there, I did it anyway.

Looking back, it may have been a necessary step in my healing process, but this blood clot didn't let me stay there for long. Its message seemed to be that it didn't matter what I had been through, my future was certainly not guaranteed. When your health is challenged, you unconsciously make all kinds of bargains. I guess somewhere inside I mistakenly thought, or at least *hoped*, my surgery had *earned* me a future.

I was certain that my own death was already in the forefront of my mind, but it seemed that keeping it there was like trying to hold a freshly caught rainbow trout in my hands. It's slippery and just keeps wiggling away. The possibility of my death took center stage in my life once again, but I noticed that I was not as shocked or frightened as when this all began.

Putting "Cancer" to Rest

My blood clot eventually resolved itself and was reabsorbed into my body. It did cloud my recovery for several months as I struggled with blood thinning medications that left me nauseous and exhausted. The clot kept me intimately plugged into the medical world, this time more locally, and brought a confrontation with the word I had avoided throughout my entire treatment, the word *cancer*.

My doctors here in my rural community didn't seem to understand that calling LAMN cancer was controversial, so I was forced to learn to dance with that scary word and all the discomfort associated with it. I was surprised when my internist put me on blood thinners saying, "Because of your cancer, this clot is more concerning." She referred to my cancer several times. My stomach did a little flip, and my chest tightened each time I heard that word. After several other references, I did tell her that Dr. Adam didn't use the word cancer in referring to my disease. I was met with an uncomfortable silence.

When the internist left her practice, she referred me to the hematology clinic at our local hospital for follow-up. "Are you coming here for your cancer or your blood clot?" the receptionist asked when scheduling my appointment. I couldn't escape that word! The doctors there kept referring to my cancer as well. At one point I checked back in with Dr. Adam's office. "You have a surgical disease. You do not have cancer. You have neoplasms," they told me. But each time I told that to my local doctors, it seemed they were thinking, *Poor dear, she is in denial.* I wasn't just imagining this because I even got a little lecture on denial from one of the practitioners. Dr. Adam offered to call my doctors. "They need educating," he told me. But I declined because that would be too big a job, contacting the rolling cast of characters that come and go here. Such is rural medicine. He suggested I get a second opinion about the blood thinners and referred me to a hematologist at UCSF.

I was able to meet with the UCSF doctor remotely. After talking with me, he told me it was okay to stop the blood thinners, but in the conversation he mentioned my "cancer."

"Dr. Adam doesn't call what I have cancer," I told him. "Well, I hate to burst your bubble, but you do, you have cancerous neoplasms." It wasn't just my rural doctors who weren't up to speed.

At that point I decided to surrender. The word *cancer* was not going to disappear, so I decided I had to defang it for myself. It was too big a job for Dr. Adam, a specialist in my disease, to educate the rest of the medical world and definitely too big a job for me.

With my new mindset, I went to my dentist. He is always friendly, but I hate dental work. I'm not that open when I go there. My dentist asked me how I'd been. I told him I'd had a medical crisis, and then I said it right out loud, without any hesitation. "I have appendiceal cancer. I had a huge surgery last fall." I felt the word *cancer* fill the entire treatment room. What power! When I got up to leave, I was startled when he gave me a huge bear hug—not our usual way of relating.

When I left the dentist office, I sat in my car for a moment trying to take in all that had just happened. That was the first and the last time I spoke in that way. Cancer is too big a word. It is like a bomb going off. It leaves a big hole. It leaves people wondering if they will ever see you again. I know it can bring forward caring and concern, but I've also seen how it makes some people run away.

In my small town I never make a trip to the grocery store or the post office without running into people I've known in one way or another over all the years I've lived here. Rumor spreads quickly through our town, and many had heard about my surgery. Now when people ask if I'm okay, I explain about the neoplasms that grew in my abdomen. I tell them I'm good now and will more than likely die of something else. That is what feels comfortable for me, but as those words come out of my mouth, I feel a little twinge of survivor guilt. There are others who live with cancer—the word, the illness, and the treatments. I feel like they are my sisters and my brothers.

Reviewing My Life

Placing my death center stage in my life again brought a surprise. I began to notice, quite spontaneously, that a life review was bubbling up into my consciousness. I found myself recalling moments over my lifetime when I had fallen short of my good intentions. Some of the memories were of gross mistakes, others of small insensitivities. All were moments when I had strayed from the path I had set out for myself. I suppose in a Christian sense, they qualified as sins.

Years ago, a former therapist had told me that the word "sin" in the Jewish tradition can be best understood as "missing the mark," an old archery term for when an arrow fails to meet its target. I've always found that interpretation wonderfully comforting, as it suggests that in our actions we were aiming for the center, but for whatever reason, missed it. The road to forgiveness is more easily traveled when we think of sin as simply having missed the mark, rather than being evil intentioned and purposefully uncaring.

It might sound as if these memories of mistakes, large and small, were the voice of my inner critic, but it wasn't like that. Instead, such memories were grounded in a deep sense of compassion for myself. As each memory presented itself, I saw what went wrong, the pain caused, and my lack of consciousness. As I sat with each one, I could see that I had clearly missed an opportunity to be more aware, more loving. It wasn't that I had done something terribly wrong, rather that I had missed the mark in letting my loving heart guide me. There was sadness in witnessing the missed opportunity, but I was not despicable. I was simply a work in progress.

If I had been a Catholic, I might, over the years, have confessed these sins to my priest and asked for absolution. As someone who grew up in a church that didn't have that ritual, I had always thought it would be a handy way to deal with the parts of us that go astray. My life review reminded me of the ritual of confession, but now, in this review, my own compassionate heart stood in for the priest, and I seemed to be absolving myself as I went along. Love was at the center of this process, rather than penance or punishment.

I recalled the biblical teaching that when we die, we meet Saint Peter at the Pearly Gates. Your life is reviewed, and it is then determined (rather heartlessly) whether you go to Heaven or Hell. This used to terrify me as a child, even though I was a very, very good little girl. Now I saw it as the Church's attempt to control by doling out rewards and punishments, not trusting that we each have a barometer inside ourselves that knows on some level when our hearts are open and when they are closed.

Paper Cranes for Peace and Love

As these memories continued to arise, I wanted to honor the process in some way. I created what I now see as a purification ritual that helped me to hold the old Marilyn in my heart as I let go of her and welcomed my new life. I decided to fold a paper crane for each one of my memories. I had not done origami before but was drawn to making cranes because they were a symbol of peace. My life review seemed an experience of internal peacemaking.

It turned out that it wasn't as easy to make the cranes as I had thought. I laughed as I replayed the instructional video on YouTube, over and over again. I folded and unfolded, trying to master the steps. More than one piece of paper became creased every which way but didn't end up looking at all like a crane. It was a study in imperfection and a time to marvel at my incompetence, a message that mirrored my life review.

Even as I got better at doing it, I folded one entire crane with the brightly colored side of the paper completely on the inside. I somehow thought that in the process, one fold or another would magically turn it inside out, which of course it didn't. That crane symbolized the radical introversion of my young life, when I didn't really recognize the beautiful color of my own soul and thus didn't have the confidence to bring the best of me out into the world.

The whole process began to feel like a metaphor for life, how when we are trying to learn something, we miss the mark again and again until we come closer and closer to who we want to be. That process never ends, as there is always more to learn. There is no way to master the art of becoming a loving human being.

I hadn't realized that my idea to make a crane for each of my moments of "missing the mark" would teach me so much, that it would remind me of how integral the process of trying things out and failing is to our becoming. We are a process, not a product. We are in a constant state of unfolding until the day we die, and then none of us knows what happens next.

I'm not sure you can find your way to being the best of yourself if you can't also know and accept the worst of who you are. Years ago, when I first began to open to the shadowy parts of myself in therapy, I remember arriving home from a session, crawling into bed, and pulling the covers over my head. I wasn't sure I would get up again. It was perhaps the closest I have come to feeling suicidal. Now, here I was holding all those parts of me in a loving embrace. If my companionship with my own death was bringing this much love and self-acceptance my way, I wanted to cultivate that relationship. Loving myself seemed at the root of loving others. I was clearly making peace with myself through this process. I've always thought being at peace with oneself was an important place to start in the desire for peace in our world. It is the one place we actually have a lot of control.

As I placed each finished crane, the beautiful ones and the malformed imperfect ones, into a basket that formed a little nest, I made wishes and whispered, "May I deepen my awareness of the present moment. May I let my open heart be my guide."

I felt the circle of life turning inside me as my conscious brushes with death passed me by and delivered me once again from winter to spring in my life. Symbolically, we die many times over in our lives as we move from one stage to another, leaving our old self behind and stepping into who we have become.

As I have come out the other side of this healing journey, the new Marilyn is becoming palpable and real to me at last. I've made a vitally important discovery that stands me in good stead no matter how long I may yet have to live. I feel more loved than I have every felt in my entire life. I do not imagine that the amount of the love coming my way has radically changed, rather I'm simply more able to receive it. This has changed my life in a myriad of ways. If my illness and my surgery have delivered me back into the world with more capacity to love and be loved, it was worth everything I have experienced.

Touching Two Worlds

As life moved forward, I realized I had exhausted myself with all my fears and questions about my own ending. It seemed I no longer had the energy to ride up and down on that roller coaster of emotions. One day, in the simple way my deeper self uses to communicate with me, a childhood song popped into my mind and wouldn't let go. The lyric, "*Que sera, sera*, whatever will be, will be, the future's not ours to see, *que sera, sera*," rolled round and round in my mind for days. I mark that as the time of my surrender in this whole affair. It brought me back to those two responses I held simultaneously when I went into surgery: *I want more life*, and *if I die, I die.* That will be okay. I found current relevance in that realization.

I have lived a full and beautiful life, beautiful not because it has been all joy and light, but because I learned to dive into the depths of all that life has brought my way. I have experienced the light and the dark and everything in between. While I haven't manifested everything I might like to manifest, I won't die regretting an unlived life. There is great peace in that thought. I have often heard that our fear of death is really our fear of life coming to us in disguise. With that thought, I'm ready now to tip the scales toward life. As I go forward, I'll be asking *What is in me that yet wants to be lived?*

At the very same time, I do not want to forget the lessons I've learned as I brushed up against death through this passage. One day, the words of a Rumi poem popped into my head and repeated throughout the day: *Don't go back to sleep.* I heard it like a mantra throughout that whole day. Unfortunately, my body took those words literally that night as I woke up at 2:00 a.m. and didn't go back to sleep for the rest of the night. That struck me as very funny when I realized it days later. Our bodies are so concrete in their way of thinking.

Here is the verse from Rumi's poem "The Breeze at Dawn."

The breeze at dawn has secrets to tell you.
Don't go back to sleep.
You must ask for what you really want.
Don't go back to sleep.
People are going back and forth across the doorsill
where the two worlds touch.
The door is round and open.
Don't go back to sleep.

–from *The Essential Rumi*, translated by Coleman Barks

I have gone "back and forth across the doorsill where the two worlds touch" again and again throughout this healing journey. My dreams, my imagination, and my art have helped me to do that. Their magic lets me see that there is more to this life I am living than meets the eye. I can't explain it. I don't even want to name it, but the love and the peace that I find when "the two worlds touch" sustains me. That love and peace held me through this time of great need. It is there for all of us. "The door is round and open."

Blessings on your journey.

Now It's Your Turn

We all have our own ways of looking within, but if you would like to experiment with some of mine you can find ideas for creative ways to reflect on themes from each of the chapters in my book on my website. You will find suggestions for experiences in artmaking, body awareness, movement, poetry and journal writing. Whether you are facing serious illness or some other kind of disruption, these activities will help you open to your imagination, explore new possibilities for responding to your situation, and put you in touch with your own deepest wisdom.

My suggestions can be enjoyed on your own. As I've said in my book, we are all creative. It comes with being human. So go for it! If you would like a mentor for your creative exploration, I am available for creative sessions in person and by video conferencing. You can contact me at www.marilynhagar.com.

Thank you for reading my book all the way to the very end! I hope it has triggered your imagination in ways that are supportive to your healing journey. I wish you well in all of your inner explorations.

Many Blessings, Marilyn

Afterword

Books end but thankfully life goes on. In recent months I've found myself revisiting the word cancer and how I am relating to it. When I was first diagnosed I'll admit that I was relieved when Dr. Adam explained that there was debate about whether to call LAMN, my disease, cancer. The whole thing was such a shock, I willingly took shelter in the comfort that his words brought. But I am a long way down the road with my disease now and am ready to let go of the fine points of how to talk about it.

I recently discovered the Appendix Cancer Pseudomyxoma Peritonei Research Foundation (ACPMP) It was created in 2008 by a community of individuals affected by the cluster of diseases bundled under the name of appendiceal cancer, LAMN among them. The foundation is dedicated to funding and supporting research to find cures. In addition they host educational programs for physicians and patients. Their website if full of useful information.

Appendiceal cancers are rare with only a 1% occurrence in the United States. With all the debate about how to classify LAMN, I hadn't really realized that I was feeling alone with this rare disease. Finding that I am a part of a much larger community has been a great gift. The day I found them, I watched several of their educational videos and read some of the patient stories on their site. When I turned off my computer I found myself buoyed by the information and the spirit of the people telling their stories. Feeling in community has helped and I now see it as an important part of my healing journey. It was heartening to learn that research is ongoing and that there are good people out there dedicating their life energy to finding cures.

The research funding from the National Institutes of Health is distributed according to the percentage of people with a particular disease so resources are small for Appendiceal cancers. You can read more and donate to the ACPMP Foundation here. https://acpmp.org.

Acknowledgments

My healing journey has left me acutely aware of how I am held by so many in this web that is life. Lives are not lived and books are not written without enormous support. I'm so grateful for all the help I have received. Many thanks…

To Joan Stanford for your enthusiastic embrace of my creative process through this healing time and for your never ending encouragement to put my story out into the world. You fed me, body and soul, through the writing of this book.

To Joanna Wigginton. Joanna thank you for your unflagging support though my entire adult life. You helped me birth babies and are now helping me birth books. Your real world support, far beyond the call of duty, is a gift beyond measure. Old friends are a treasure.

To Lindsay Wansbury. Thanks for your supportive presence through thick and thin. Your enthusiastic support of my first draft helped me take my next steps. And a huge thank you for giving me the idea to add "and the Pen" to my title.

To Tansy Chapman. Thank you for your wise woman quips, your advice about writing, your sense of humor and though we don't always agree, for our discussions about all things spiritual.

To Mary Cavagnaro and Beverly Parish for our discussions around the breakfast table. They always bring insight. They deepened my thought process about many of the topics in my book. Your early suggestions were essential.

To Sharon Hansen for all the delicious food you brought to help me heal and for offering specific and heartfelt response to my first draft. To Tom Wodetski for asking important questions and bringing your editorial skill to my project. To Laura Peritore, your helpful suggestions improved key parts of my book immensely. To Randy Bancroft for your technology advice and you kind words. To Lisa Hafner for all your good wishes during this healing time and for cheering me on with my writing. To my early readers, Leslie Lebeau, Carol Wilder, and Maria Gonzales Blue for your time and encouragement. To my childhood friend Judy Espiau for reconnecting so lovingly through this healing time and for being my co-conspirator in all our "Let's pretend" games as children.

To my women's group. Thank you Cornelia Gerken, Tracey Coddington, Sidra Stone, and Sharon Hansen for witnessing my life journey and holding me so lovingly through this healing time. Your early reading of my first draft and your enthusiasm about my creative process encourages me onward.

To my dream group. Thank you Larry Sawyer, Harriet Bye, Tom Wodetski, Sharon Hansen, Cornelia Gerkin, Kris Reiber, Tansy Chapman, and Pat Ferrero for sharing dreams with me all these years. You have enriched my inner life in a multitude of ways with your dreams, your insights and your impressions.

To Michael Meade, thank you for giving me permission to use the story of The Old Woman of the World here, and to Coleman Barks thank you for allowing me to use your translation of the Rumi poem "The Breeze at Dawn" in this book. I thank both of you for your generosity.

To Brook Warner and She Writes Press for giving me the idea that at this late stage in life, I could be an author. I doubt that I would have ever thought to write this book if you had not mentored me so thoughtfully through the process of publishing *Finding the Wild Inside.*

To Annie Tucker my editor for *Finding the Wild Inside.* Your voice is alive inside of me all these years later. We carried on many conversation inside my own head as I wrote this new book. I can't thank you enough for all your help. Your teachings were inspiring and have deeply enriched my writing life.

To my editor Nancy Marriott at New Paradigm Literary Services. You had a sharp eye for details but also the ability to grasp the big picture of my book. You were always thinking about my readers and how they might be responding or not responding in the way I intended. You helped me strengthen my voice and bring clarity and focus to my message. Thank you Nancy.

To Cynthia Frank at Cypress House. Thank you for guiding me through all the hoops so that *The Scalpel, The Paintbrush, and the Pen* can quickly find its way out into the world. Your support and expertise has been a great gift. Thank you to your team, Joe, Allegra and Susan for your important contributions along the way. Very much appreciated.

To Carla Stange. I will be forever grateful for your medical expertise and for sending me down to UCSF. Thank you for being willing to read my book and for considering making a comment.

To Dr. Mohamed Adam. Without your help I may not have been here to see this book enter the world. My story would have been very different without your skill, your openness and your caring. There aren't enough words to express my gratitude. You promised that you and your team would be "all in" to help me through my surgery and you were that big time.

Thanks to Stacy Alabastro, NP for calming my jitters about the OR and for your continued medical support, Michelle Irner, RN BSN for your help in preparing for surgery and your answers to so many questions, and to Jessi Dailey for your welcoming voice on the phone and for shepherding me through the system at UCSF, making appointments, scheduling tests etc. And a big thank you to all those at the hospital whose names I don't recall. I couldn't have had a better experience (before, during and after my surgery) than I have had at UCSF.

To the most important people in my life, my family. Thank you Erik, Kristiann, Andrew, Alex, Gabriel, Stacy, Chase, Cole, Eli and Amy for your enormous support during my healing time. I couldn't have felt more loved. Eli, thank you for your advice about my subtitle and to all of you, your enthusiasm, and your real world support for my writing has been a great gift and is very much appreciated.

About the Author

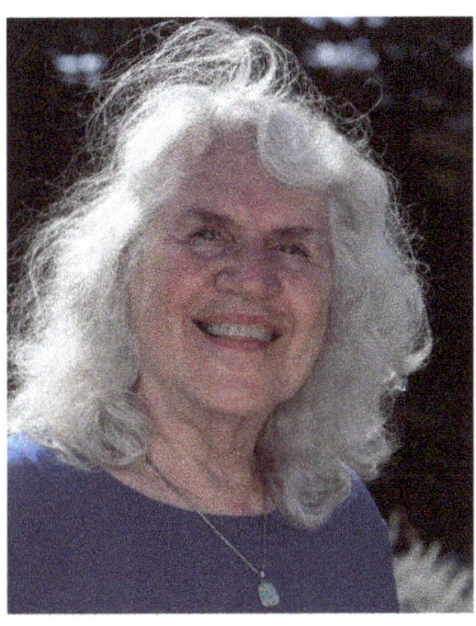

Marilyn Hagar is a registered expressive arts therapist and author of *Finding the Wild Inside: Exploring Our Inner Landscape Through the Arts, Dreams, and Intuition.* She believes that expressing ourselves through the arts broadens our perspective and puts us in touch with our deepest inner wisdom. When Marilyn was diagnosed with a rare form of cancer, her intuition, her dreams, and the arts became her trusted companions on her healing journey. She wants us all to know that these ways of looking within are available to everyone. We are all creative—it comes with being human. Marilyn is available to speak to groups about empowering ourselves as patients by finding our wise healer within. She leads personal creative retreats at For the Joy of It in Mendocino, California.

Visit www.marilynhagar.com.